Fast Facts

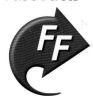

Fast Facts:
Chronic Obstructive
Pulmonary Disease

DATE DUE

D FRCP
onmental Medicine

chool

icine Section

enter

cts.com

HEALTH PRESS

Fast Facts: Chronic Obstructive Pulmonary Disease
First published 2004
Second edition August 2009

Text © 2009 William MacNee, Stephen I Rennard
© 2009 in this edition Health Press Limited
Health Press Limited, Elizabeth House, Queen Street, Abingdon,
Oxford OX14 3LN, UK
Tel: +44 (0)1235 523233
Fax: +44 (0)1235 523238

Book orders can be placed by telephone or via the website.
For regional distributors or to order via the website, please go to:
www.fastfacts.com
For telephone orders, please call +44 (0)1752 202301 (UK and Europe),
1 800 247 6553 (USA, toll free), +1 419 281 1802 (Americas) or
+61 (0)2 9698 7755 (Asia–Pacific).

Fast Facts is a trademark of Health Press Limited.

A CIP record for this title is available from the British Library.

ISBN 978-1-905832-54-5

MacNee W (William)
Fast Facts: Chronic Obstructive Pulmonary Disease/
William MacNee, Stephen I Rennard

Typesetting and page layout by Zed, Oxford, UK.
Printed by Latimer Trend & Company Limited, Plymouth, UK.

Text printed on biodegradable and recyclable paper
manufactured using elemental chlorine free (ECF)
wood pulp from well-managed forests.

FSC

Mixed Sources
Product group from well-managed
forests and other controlled sources

Cert no. SGS-COC-005493
www.fsc.org
© 1996 Forest Stewardship Council

Glossary of abbreviations

BMI: body mass index

BODE index: a measure of disease severity that incorporates body mass index, obstruction, dyspnea and ability to exercise

cAMP: cyclic adenosine monophosphate

COPD: chronic obstructive pulmonary disease

CT: computed tomography

DLco: diffusing capacity in the lung for carbon monoxide (sometimes called TLco in the UK)

ECG: electrocardiography/electrocardiogram

FEV_1: forced expiratory volume in 1 second

FVC: forced vital capacity (the total volume of air that can be exhaled from a maximum inhalation to a maximum exhalation)

GOLD: Global initiative for chronic Obstructive Lung Disease

HRCT: high-resolution computed tomography

ICU: intensive care unit

IL: interleukin

Kco: carbon monoxide transfer coefficient ($DLco/V_A$)

MRC: Medical Research Council (UK)

NHLBI: National Heart, Lung and Blood Institute (USA)

NIPPV: non-invasive intermittent positive-pressure ventilation

$PaCO_2$: partial pressure of carbon dioxide in arterial blood

PaO_2: partial pressure of oxygen in arterial blood

PEF: peak expiratory flow

SaO_2: percentage oxygen saturation of arterial blood

SGRQ: St George's Respiratory Questionnaire

V_A: ventilated alveolar volume, or accessible lung volume

V_T: tidal volume

VC: vital capacity

WHO: World Health Organization

Introduction

Chronic obstructive pulmonary disease (COPD) has not always elicited sympathetic interest from the medical community. In their groundbreaking monograph on the natural history of COPD, Fletcher and colleagues chose the following quote to emphasize the self-perpetuating attitude that has unfortunately inhibited the understanding and management of COPD.

> '...medicine has come a long way since 1925, when Williams, writing *Middle Age and Old Age*, could confidently assert: "Chronic bronchitis with its accompanying emphysema is a disease on which a good deal of wholly unmerited sympathy is frequently wasted. It is a disease of the gluttonous, bibulous, otiose and obese and represents a well-deserved nemesis for these unlovely indulgences ... the majority of cases are undoubtedly due to surfeit and self-indulgence."'

Since the landmark study of Fletcher and Peto, great gains have been made in understanding the pathogenesis, physiology, clinical features and management of COPD. Cigarette smoking, itself now regarded as a disease, is the major risk factor. However, COPD also occurs in non-smokers, and individuals vary greatly in their susceptibility to smoke. Moreover, COPD is a heterogeneous collection of syndromes with overlapping manifestations. This has led to considerable variance in definitions, which has confounded epidemiological and cross-national studies. The Global initiative for chronic Obstructive Lung Disease (GOLD) was recently implemented in order to provide some uniformity. GOLD defines COPD as: 'a preventable and treatable disease with some significant extra-pulmonary effects that may contribute to the severity in individual patients. The pulmonary component is characterized by airflow limitation that is not fully reversible. The airflow limitation is usually progressive and associated with an abnormal inflammatory response of the lung to noxious particles and gases'.

COPD was estimated to be the twelfth leading cause of morbidity and the sixth leading cause of death worldwide in 1990. Of all the major diseases, COPD presents the fastest increasing healthcare burden. By 2030, mortality from COPD is predicted to more than double, accounting for more than 5.6 million deaths (Table 1). COPD patients, moreover, often make few complaints despite suffering considerable disability. As a result, although COPD can easily be diagnosed, it frequently is not.

The relationship between asthma and COPD has been particularly troublesome. Defining asthma as 'reversible' led to the inference that COPD is 'irreversible' and, therefore, that there was nothing to 'reverse' with treatment. This incorrect belief has served only to exacerbate the underdiagnosis and undertreatment of COPD. Distinguishing between

TABLE 1

Causes of death in 2002 and projected figures for 2030 ($\times 10^3$)

	Number of deaths in 2002	Projected number of deaths in 2030	Change (%)
HIV/AIDS	2853	6501	128
Diabetes mellitus	983	2207	124
COPD	2746	5684	107
Cancer	7109	11 485	62
Lung cancer	1242	2242	81
Stomach cancer	850	1389	64
Hypertensive heart disease	908	1338	47
Neuropsychiatric disorders	1109	1627	47
Intentional injuries	1614	2292	42
Stroke	5502	7788	42
Ischemic heart disease	7195	9843	37
Accidents/unintentional injuries	3545	4796	35
Digestive diseases	1964	2325	18
Respiratory infections	4018	2617	−35
Perinatal conditions	2459	1577	−36

AIDS, acquired immunodeficiency syndrome; HIV, human immunodeficiency virus.
Data from Mathers and Loncar, 2006.

asthma and COPD can be difficult. Both conditions are associated with chronic airway inflammation, although the underlying chronic inflammation is very different in each disease. Both conditions can occur in the same individual and some patients with asthma may progress to COPD, even in the absence of smoking. The clinical problem, however, is not whether a patient has asthma or COPD, but rather whether either asthma or COPD is present, or both.

COPD is associated with a number of comorbidities. While most are common conditions, they are seen more frequently in patients with COPD than would normally be expected. This has led to the concept that COPD has systemic effects, perhaps due to an underlying chronic inflammatory process. Often these comorbidities present major clinical problems in the individual patient for whom the recognition and treatment of COPD is key to management.

COPD is a very expensive disorder. Costs in the USA are estimated to be nearly $40 billion annually; two-thirds of these costs are direct and one-third indirect. Since COPD is significantly underdiagnosed, these estimates are likely to be highly conservative. Most costs associated with COPD are due to exacerbations, particularly those that result in hospitalization. Since exacerbations increase in frequency and require a greater level of care as COPD progresses, most costs are incurred towards the end stage of the disease. General healthcare costs are also increased in COPD patients, emphasizing the multisystem problems faced by this patient group.

Previous guidelines have emphasized treatment for patients who have lost 50–65% of their lung function. Recent guidelines, however, recognize that diagnosis and treatment of COPD at earlier stages can have substantial benefits for the patient. While currently available treatments are unable to cure COPD, they can reduce symptoms, improve lung function and reduce exacerbations, and may decrease the healthcare costs associated with the disease. In addition, treatment may slow the rate of decline in lung function and has demonstrable effects on mortality that approach statistical significance.

Key references

Fletcher C, Peto R. The natural history of chronic airflow obstruction. *BMJ* 1977;1:1645–8.

Fletcher C, Peto R, Tinker C, Speizer FE. *The Natural History of Chronic Bronchitis and Emphysema: An Eight-Year Study of Early Chronic Obstructive Lung Disease in Working Men in London.* New York: Oxford University Press, 1976:1–272.

Global initiative for chronic Obstructive Lung Disease. *Global Strategy for the Diagnosis, Management, and Prevention of Chronic Obstructive Pulmonary Disease. NHLBI/WHO Workshop Report.* Updated 2008. www.goldcopd.com/Guidelineitem .asp?l1=2&l2=1&intId=2003 Accessed 12 January 2009.

Mathers CD, Loncar D. Projections of global mortality and burden of disease from 2002 to 2030. *PLoS Med* 2006;3:e442.

Shapiro SD, Snider GL, Rennard SI. Chronic bronchitis and emphysema. In: Mason RJ, Broadus VC, Murray JF, Nadel JA, eds. *Textbook of Respiratory Medicine.* 4th edn. Philadelphia: Elsevier, 2005:1115–67.

1 Pathology and pathogenesis

In COPD, pathological changes occur in the central conducting airways, the peripheral airways, the lung parenchyma and the pulmonary vasculature. Inflammation induced by cigarette smoke underlies most pathological lesions associated with COPD. Inflammation also contributes to recurrent exacerbations of COPD, in which acute inflammation is superimposed on the chronic disease. There is now good evidence that all smokers develop lung inflammation; however, some individuals are more susceptible to the effects of cigarette smoke and are more severely affected. The pathogenesis of COPD in non-smokers has been less studied, but inflammation secondary to air pollution or other substances is likely to play a key role. The extent of the pathological changes in the different lung compartments varies between individuals and results in the clinical and pathophysiological heterogeneity seen in patients with COPD.

Some believe that chronic asthma should be included as part of the spectrum of COPD. Although the clinical and physiological presentation of chronic asthma may be indistinguishable from that of COPD, the pathological changes are distinct from those in most COPD cases due to cigarette smoking. Histological features of COPD in the 15–20% of COPD patients who are non-smokers have not been well studied.

Chronic bronchitis

Chronic bronchitis is defined clinically by the American Thoracic Society and the UK Medical Research Council as: 'the production of sputum on most days for at least 3 months in at least 2 consecutive years'. This chronic hypersecretion of mucus results from changes in the central airways – the trachea, bronchi and bronchioles over 2–4 mm in internal diameter. Mucus is produced by mucus glands, which are present mainly in the larger airways, and by goblet cells, found in the airway epithelium.

In chronic bronchitis, hypertrophy of mucus glands occurs mainly in the larger bronchi and is associated with infiltration of the glands by inflammatory cells (Figure 1.1). In healthy never-smokers, goblet cells

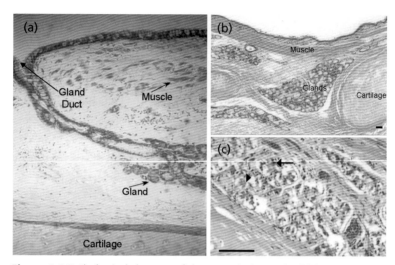

Figure 1.1 Pathological changes of the central airways in COPD.
(a) A central bronchus from the lungs of a cigarette smoker with normal function shows small amounts of muscle present in the subepithelium and small epithelial glands. (b) In a patient with chronic bronchitis, the muscle appears as a thick bundle and the bronchial glands are enlarged.
(c) At a higher magnification, these glands show evidence of a chronic inflammatory process involving polymorphonuclear leukocytes (arrowhead) and mononuclear cells, including plasma cells (arrow). Reproduced from the Global Initiative for Chronic Obstructive Lung Disease Workshop 2001, Original Report, with the kind permission of Professor James C Hogg, University of British Columbia, Canada.

make up 10% of the columnar epithelial cells in the proximal airways, but their numbers decrease in more distal airways and are normally absent in the terminal or respiratory bronchioles. By contrast, in smokers, goblet cells are not only present in increased numbers but also extend more peripherally. Metaplastic or dysplastic changes in the surface epithelium may replace the goblet cells of the normal respiratory epithelium in some smokers and thus may reduce the number of goblet cells in the proximal airways. The clinical significance of these varied anatomic alterations is unknown.

Recent studies using bronchoscopy to obtain lavage and biopsy samples together with examination of spontaneous or induced sputum have provided new insights into the role of inflammation in COPD. Studies have reported increased numbers of neutrophils in the intraluminal space in patients with stable COPD. Bronchial biopsy studies have described inflammation in the bronchi of patients with chronic bronchitis with and without airway obstruction, and have shown that activated T lymphocytes are prominent in the proximal airways. Macrophages are also a prominent feature and, in contrast to asthma, the CD8 suppressor T-lymphocyte subset predominates in chronic bronchitis rather than the CD4 helper subset. Neutrophils are present, particularly in the glands, and become more prominent as the disease progresses.

Bronchial biopsies taken from patients during mild exacerbations of chronic bronchitis indicate increased numbers of eosinophils in the bronchial wall, though far fewer than are present in exacerbations of asthma; increased numbers of neutrophils are also observed. Eosinophils may not be prominent in severe exacerbations.

Several studies using bronchoalveolar lavage or, more recently, using spontaneous or induced sputum, have demonstrated intraluminal inflammation in the airspaces of patients with chronic bronchitis with or without airway obstruction. In stable chronic bronchitis, the high percentage of intraluminal neutrophils is associated with the presence of neutrophil chemotactic factors, including interleukin-8 (IL-8) and leukotriene B4, and other inflammatory mediators. There is also evidence that the airspace inflammation in patients with chronic bronchitis persists following smoking cessation if the production of sputum persists, though cough and sputum are reduced in most smokers who quit.

Chronic inflammation of the bronchial wall is also associated with connective tissue changes that include increased amounts of smooth muscle and degenerative changes in the airway cartilage as well as increased vascularity.

Small-airways disease/bronchiolitis

The smaller bronchi and bronchioles less than 2 mm in diameter are a major site of airway obstruction in COPD. Inflammation in the small airways is one of the earliest changes in asymptomatic cigarette smokers, and considerable changes in these airways can occur without giving rise to symptoms or alteration in spirometry measurements. Thus, this region in the lung is often referred to as the 'silent zone'. The pattern of inflammatory cell changes in the small airways resembles that in the larger airways, including the predominance of CD8+ lymphocytes and the increase in the CD8:CD4 ratio.

The mechanisms leading to the increase in peripheral airway resistance include several distinct processes: destruction of alveolar support, loss of elastic recoil in the parenchyma that contributes to this support and provides driving pressure for alveolar emptying, and structural narrowing of the airway lumen. The lumen may be occluded by mucus and cells. Mucosal ulceration, goblet cell hyperplasia and squamous cell metaplasia may be present in addition to fibrosis and mesenchymal cell accumulation. As the condition progresses, structural remodeling may occur, characterized by increased collagen content and formation of scar tissue, which narrows the airways and produces fixed airway obstruction (Figure 1.2).

Pulmonary emphysema

Pulmonary emphysema is defined in structural and pathological terms as "abnormal permanent enlargement of airspaces distal to the terminal bronchioles accompanied by destruction of their walls". The terms used to describe emphysema are based on the anatomy of the normal lung, where a secondary lobule is defined as that part of the lung that contains several terminal bronchioles surrounded by connective tissue septa. An acinus is that part of the lung parenchyma supplied by a single terminal bronchiole. Therefore, each secondary lobule contains several terminal bronchioles and thus several acini.

Emphysema is classified by the pattern of the enlarged airspaces on the cut surface of the fixed inflated lung (Figure 1.3). Airspace enlargement can be identified macroscopically when the size of the airspace reaches 1 mm. Absence of obvious fibrosis is a prerequisite in most definitions of emphysema; histologically, however, fibrosis has been recognized in the region of the terminal or respiratory bronchioles as part of a respiratory bronchiolitis that occurs in smokers, and lung collagen content is increased in mild emphysema. Three principal types of emphysema are recognized according to the distribution of the enlarged airspaces within

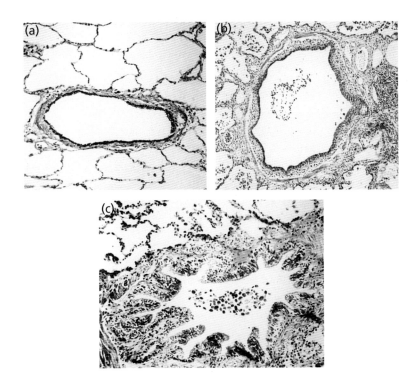

Figure 1.2 Histological sections of peripheral airways. (a) Section from a cigarette smoker with normal lung function showing a nearly normal airway. (b) Section from a patient with small-airways disease showing inflammatory exudate in the wall and lumen of the airway. (c) Section showing more advanced small-airways disease with reduced lumen, structural reorganization of the airway wall, increased smooth muscle and deposition of peribronchiolar connective tissue. Images reproduced with the kind permission of Professor James C Hogg, University of British Columbia, Canada.

the acinar unit (Figure 1.4): centriacinar (centrilobular), panacinar (panlobular) and, the least common, periacinar (paraseptal) emphysema. Other, less common forms may also occur.

Centriacinar and panacinar emphysema can occur alone or in combination. Whether the two types represent different disease processes and thus have different etiologies, or whether panacinar emphysema is a progression from centriacinar emphysema is still subject

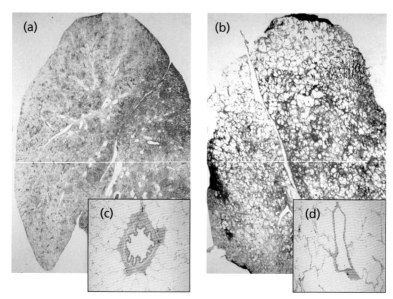

Figure 1.3 (a) Paper-mounted whole lung section of a normal lung.
(b) Paper-mounted whole lung section from a lung with severe centrilobular emphysema; note that the centrilobular form is more extensive in the upper regions of the lung. (c) Histological section of normal small airway and surrounding alveoli connecting with attached alveolar walls. (d) Histological section showing emphysema with enlarged alveolar spaces, loss of alveolar wall and attachments, and collapsed airways.

to debate. The association with cigarette smoking is certainly clearer for centriacinar than panacinar emphysema, though smokers can develop both types. Those with centriacinar emphysema appear to have more abnormalities in their small airways than those with predominantly panacinar emphysema.

Centriacinar emphysema is characterized by initial clustering of the enlarged airspaces around the terminal bronchiole. It is more prominent in the upper zones of the upper and lower lobes, and is the type most commonly seen in smokers.

Panacinar emphysema. The enlarged airspaces are distributed throughout the acinar unit. The destruction of the acinus is more uniform, and all of the acini within the secondary lobule are involved. In contrast to centriacinar emphysema, panacinar emphysema appears to be

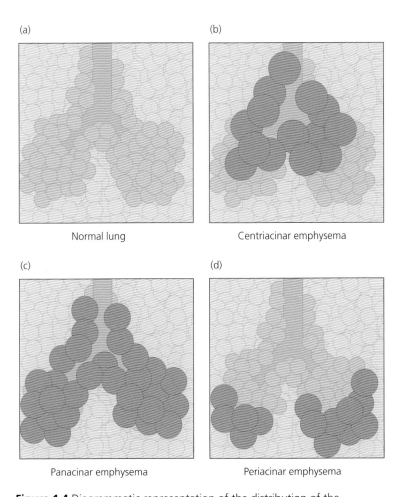

(a)

(b)

Normal lung

Centriacinar emphysema

(c)

(d)

Panacinar emphysema

Periacinar emphysema

Figure 1.4 Diagrammatic representation of the distribution of the abnormal airspaces within the acinar unit in the three major types of emphysema. (a) Acinar unit in a normal lung (although the illustration shows a clearly defined area for the purposes of clarity, it must be remembered that adjacent acinar units intercommunicate and are not necessarily demarcated by septa). (b) Centriacinar (centrilobular) emphysema: focal enlargement of the airspaces around the respiratory bronchiole. (c) Panacinar (panlobular) emphysema: confluent, even involvement of the acinar unit. (d) Periacinar (paraseptal) emphysema: peripherally distributed enlarged airspaces where the acinar unit abuts a fixed structure, such as the pleura.

15

more severe in the lower lobe, but can be found anywhere in the lungs. It is associated with α_1-proteinase inhibitor deficiency, but it can also be found in cases where no clear-cut genetic abnormality has been identified.

Periacinar (paraseptal or distal acinar) emphysema is characterized by enlargement of the airspaces along the edge of the acinar unit, but only where it abuts a fixed structure, such as the pleura or a vessel. Periacinar emphysema is usually of little clinical significance unless it occurs extensively in a subpleural position, when it may be associated with pneumothorax.

Unilateral emphysema or McLeod syndrome occurs as a complication of severe childhood infections with rubella or adenovirus.

Congenital lobular emphysema is a developmental abnormality affecting newborn children.

Scar or irregular emphysema comprises enlarged airspaces around the margins of a scar unrelated to the structure of the acinus.

Bullae are localized areas of emphysema that are overdistended. Conventionally, only lesions over 1 cm in size are described as bullae. Bullae arise in areas of lung that have been locally destroyed, though this destruction does not have to be a result of emphysema; the damage can also result from lytic or traumatic causes. They have been described in patients with tuberculosis, sarcoidosis, acquired immunodeficiency syndrome (AIDS) and trauma. The origins of bullae remain obscure. In the minority of cases, around 20%, the surrounding lung is normal, but most bullae are associated with more generalized emphysema and chronic airway obstruction.

Pulmonary vasculature

The development of chronic alveolar hypoxia in patients with COPD produces characteristic remodeling of the pulmonary arteries. However, other changes occur earlier in the natural history of the disease; the first is thickening of the intima, followed by an increase in the amount of smooth muscle and infiltration of the vessel wall with inflammatory cells. As the disease progresses, the amounts of smooth muscle, proteoglycans and collagen present in the vessel wall increase and cause it to thicken. Right ventricular hypertrophy and pulmonary hypertension are commonly found in patients with COPD who have chronic hypoxemia.

Physiological significance

The pathological changes in patients with COPD are complex and may occur to varying extents in the large and small airways, and in the alveolar compartment. It is difficult to determine clinically or by respiratory function tests the relative contributions made to airway obstruction by the different pathological changes. In general, it is thought that the smaller bronchi and bronchioles less than 2 mm in diameter are the major sites of airway obstruction in COPD.

Narrowing of small airways can result from the formation of peribronchiolar scars and consequent contraction. Consistent with this, decreased airway circumference correlates well with airflow limitation in patients with moderately severe COPD when assessed on specimens removed surgically. Emphysema leads to decreased expiratory airflow by different mechanisms. Loss of elastic recoil of the lungs decreases the driving pressure that empties the alveoli and reduces the intraluminal pressure within the terminal airways. Because of this and because of destruction of alveolar attachments that tether the small airways in an open position, small airways can collapse during forced exhalation, resulting in effort-independent limitation of expiratory airflow. Hyperinflation of the lungs with overdistension of alveoli may also lead to airway compression. Intraluminal accumulation of secretions and cells may also play a role. Symptoms and physiological abnormalities in a given individual may be due to different combinations of lesions at different stages.

The normal inflammatory response in the lungs resulting from the inhalation of irritants, such as cigarette smoke, appears to be enhanced and abnormally persistent in COPD patients. The factors responsible for the amplification of inflammation in COPD are not fully understood, but may involve genetic mechanisms. Oxidative stress, caused by an excess of oxidants in relation to antioxidants, results from the increase in oxidants inhaled in cigarette smoke, though the release of oxidants from inflammatory cells may also enhance the inflammatory response through the activation of inflammatory genes. Oxidants also inactivate protective antiproteases and cause mucus hypersecretion.

There is good evidence that an imbalance between protease release and antiproteases exists in the lungs in COPD patients which leads to the breakdown of connective tissue components in the lung parenchyma, resulting in the tissue destruction seen in emphysema.

Key points – pathology and pathogenesis

- COPD results from pathological changes in the large and small airways (bronchiolitis) and in the alveolar space (emphysema).
- Chronic bronchitis is defined clinically as the production of sputum on most days for at least 3 months a year over at least 2 consecutive years.
- Inflammation occurs in large and small airways, and in the alveolar space, involving a number of cells including neutrophils, macrophages and T lymphocytes, particularly CD8+ lymphocytes.
- Small-airways disease or bronchiolitis can result in inflammation and eventually scarring of the small airways; this is an important pathological change in COPD, which is difficult to assess by respiratory function tests, but may be a major source of airway obstruction.
- Centriacinar emphysema is the most common form of emphysema, which occurs particularly in smokers, and is distributed mainly in the upper zones of the lungs. Panacinar emphysema has a more diffuse distribution with a predominance in the lower zones of the lungs, and is associated with α_1-antitrypsin deficiency but can also occur in some smokers.
- Bullae are emphysematous spaces over 1 cm in diameter.
- Combinations of these pathological changes occur to varying degrees in different individuals with COPD and contribute to the airflow limitation.
- The lungs of COPD patients show an amplified and persistent inflammatory response to the inhalation of particles and gases, particularly those in cigarette smoke. A protease:antiprotease and oxidant:antioxidant imbalance is part of this amplified inflammatory response.

Key references

Chung KF, Adcock IM. Multifaceted mechanisms in COPD: inflammation, immunity, and tissue repair and destruction. *Eur Respir J* 2008; 31:1334–56.

Global Initiative for Chronic Obstructive Lung Disease. Pathogenesis, pathology, and pathophysiology. *Global Strategy for the Diagnosis, Management, and Prevention of Chronic Obstructive Pulmonary Disease. NHLBI/WHO Workshop Report.* Updated 2008. www.goldcopd.com/Guidelineitem .asp?l1=2&l2=1&intId=2003 Accessed 12 January 2009.

Global Initiative for Chronic Obstructive Lung Disease. *2001 Original: Workshop Report, Global Strategy for Diagnosis, Management, and Prevention of COPD.* www.goldcopd.com/Guidelineitem .asp?l1=2&l2=1&intId=1151 Accessed 3 March 2009.

Hogg JC. The pathophysiology of airflow limitation in chronic obstructive pulmonary disease. *Lancet* 2004;364:709–21.

Hogg JC, Timens W. The pathology of chronic obstructive pulmonary disease. *Annu Rev Pathol* 2008; Oct 27 [Epub ahead of print].

MacNee W. The pathogenesis of chronic obstructive pulmonary disease. *Clin Chest Med* 2007;28:479–513.

Saetta M, Turato G, Maestrelli P et al. Cellular and structural bases of chronic obstructive pulmonary disease. *Am J Respir Crit Care Med* 2001;163:1304–9.

Saetta M, Turato G, Timens W, Geffery P. Pathology of chronic obstructive pulmonary disease. *Eur Respir Mon* 2006;38;159–76.

The measure most commonly used to monitor the natural history of COPD is forced expiratory volume in 1 second (FEV_1). This parameter can be readily measured by spirometry (see Chapter 4). Most studies of COPD have relied on FEV_1 as the key measure to assess the etiology, natural history and susceptibility of individuals to the development of the disease.

FEV_1 is justly regarded as the single most important objective measure of COPD for both research and clinical purposes. However, several other clinical parameters independently characterize the features of the disease (see Chapter 4).

Etiology

The conducting airways are fully developed by 16 weeks' gestation. Alveolar structures develop both pre- and postnatally, increasing in number in early childhood up to about the age of 8 years. Alveolar size continues to increase with lung growth. Maximal lung function is reached in young adulthood and correlates with the attainment of maximal body size. Women achieve maximal lung function sooner than men due to their earlier growth spurt and epiphyseal closures. Lung function, after reaching a maximum in young adulthood, remains stable for a decade or so and then begins to decline at a slowly increasing rate. On average, FEV_1 declines by about 20 mL/year after the age of 30, and by up to 30 mL/year by 70 years of age.

Risk factors

Cigarette smoking is the most important etiologic factor for the development of COPD. There is a highly significant dose and duration effect, with smokers having lower lung function the more and longer they smoke. There is, however, considerable individual variation. Some non-smokers, for example, have impaired lung function. Approximately 20% of COPD patients (see below) are lifelong non-smokers.

Conversely, some heavy smokers are able to maintain normal lung function (Figure 2.1).

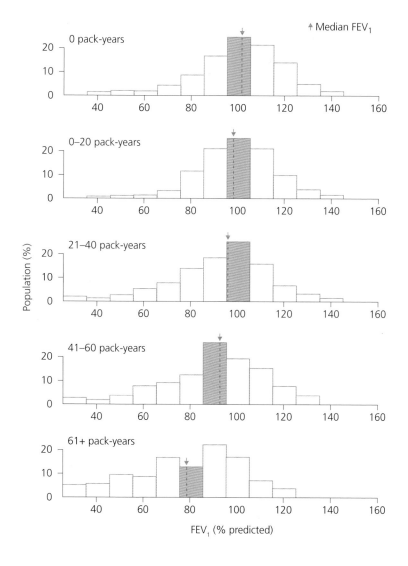

Figure 2.1 Distribution of values for forced expiratory volume in 1 second (FEV_1) expressed as a percentage of the predicted value for groups with differing smoking histories. Data from Burrows et al. 1979.

It is likely that smoking contributes to the development of COPD in several distinct ways and at several different periods over the lifespan of the individual (Table 2.1). Furthermore, the adverse effects of smoking on lung function are likely to be greater the earlier an individual is exposed.

Exposure to other substances, including indoor and outdoor pollution, can also contribute to the development of COPD. Passive exposure to cigarette smoke is an important risk and may contribute to the development of COPD in non-smokers. Individuals exposed to dusts and fumes who also smoke cigarettes have the highest risk of developing COPD.

The mechanisms by which cigarette smoke leads to COPD are under intensive study, as they offer potential opportunities for therapeutic intervention. Smoke is capable of inducing an inflammatory response through a number of mechanisms. It induces release of proinflammatory mediators from epithelial cells present in the lower respiratory tract, as well as from resident macrophages. It can also activate complement. Thus, the inflammation that is characteristically present in the lungs of

TABLE 2.1

Mechanisms by which smoking may contribute to COPD

Prenatal exposure
- Reduced lung development
- Low birth weight

Childhood
- Decreased lung growth and thus decreased maximal attained lung function

Adulthood
- Reduction in the 'plateau phase' during which lung function remains stable in young adulthood
- Accelerated onset of lung function decline
- Lung destruction
- Impaired lung repair

smokers probably results from activation of multiple pathways. The mediators released by inflammatory cells and parenchymal cells recruited and stimulated by cigarette smoke are capable of inducing lung damage. These mediators include reactive oxygen species, active proteinases and toxic peptides. In addition, cigarette smoke can decrease levels of antioxidants and antiproteinases that serve to mitigate damage caused by these toxic moieties. These effects therefore tip the balance in the lung toward tissue damage both by increasing the production of toxic mediators and by decreasing defenses.

Smoke may also alter the ability of the lungs to self-repair. This feature may resemble the widely recognized systemic adverse effect smoke has on wound healing. In other words, smoke can both increase tissue damage and impair the ability to repair that damage.

The complex interactions between cigarette smoke and the lungs of smokers suggest multiple steps at which individual susceptibility may vary. Consistent with this, smokers show considerable heterogeneity in their susceptibility to developing COPD and strong genetic components appear to be present. Both smoking and non-smoking siblings of individuals with established COPD are at greatly increased risk of lower lung function than are siblings of individuals without COPD. It is likely that a number of specific genetic factors will affect susceptibility to COPD.

Low maximal attained lung function increases the risk of excessive loss of lung function in later life. Not surprisingly, a variety of early life events can increase the risk for the development of COPD, presumably by affecting lung growth and development. Individuals with low birth weight, for example, have been shown to have both a reduced maximal attained lung function in young adult life and reduced lung function as they get older. Some childhood infections have been reported both to reduce lung function in adulthood and to increase the risk of pulmonary symptoms. Interestingly, these infections may affect lung function in several ways. In addition to acutely altering lung growth and development, some infections may have direct effects in later life. Specifically, small portions of some viral genomes can be chronically incorporated and expressed in lung cells. Such expression may predispose individuals to inflammation and lung damage in later life.

Airway hyperreactivity is also a risk factor for the development of COPD. It is measured by challenging individuals with low doses of the acetylcholine analog methacholine or with histamine. The challenge results in constriction of airway smooth muscle and a reduction in airflow, usually measured by FEV_1. A lower dose of methacholine is required to reduce airflow by 20% in hyperreactive airways than in normal airways (Figure 2.2). The fact that asthma is characterized by increased airway reactivity and individuals with increased reactivity have a greater risk of developing COPD suggests a link between asthma and COPD. Consistent with this, a proportion of patients with asthma appear to have an accelerated rate of decline in lung function suggestive of COPD.

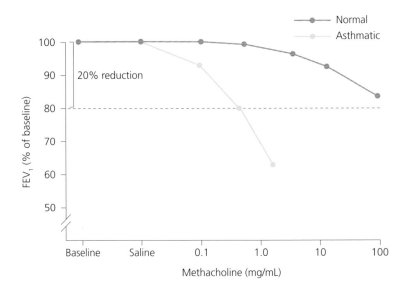

Figure 2.2 Airflow in hyperreactive airways is reduced by a lower dose of methacholine than airflow in normal airways. Here the normal and asthmatic responses to a methacholine challenge are plotted in terms of the forced expiratory volume in 1 second (FEV_1), expressed as a percentage of the baseline value, against methacholine dose. Adapted with permission from Baum GL, Crapo JD, Celli B, Karlinsky J, eds. *Textbook of Pulmonary Diseases*, 6th edn, vol I. Philadelphia: Lippincott Raven, 1998:209.

Genetic factors that are possibly related to COPD risk are listed in Table 2.2. Several candidate genes have been suggested, but to date, the only widely accepted genetic association with COPD is α_1-proteinase inhibitor deficiency (α_1-antitrypsin deficiency). People deficient in α_1-proteinase inhibitor are at increased risk of developing COPD even if they do not smoke. If such individuals smoke, they are likely to develop severe COPD at a particularly early age (Figure 2.3). α_1-proteinase inhibitor is a major inhibitor of serine proteinases, including neutrophil elastase; thus it is postulated that α_1-proteinase inhibitor deficiency results in excess activity of neutrophil elastase and therefore tissue destruction and emphysema. However, only some non-smokers with α_1-proteinase inhibitor deficiency develop emphysema. Some maintain normal lung function throughout life. This indicates the importance of other factors.

Though not yet established, it has been suggested that several other genes contribute to the development of COPD. Interestingly, many of

TABLE 2.2

Components possibly related to genetic pathogenesis of COPD

- α_1-proteinase inhibitor
- α_1-antichymotrypsin
- α_2-macroglobulin
- Serine protease inhibitor nexin 2
- Matrix metalloproteinase-1
- Matrix metalloproteinase-9
- Matrix metalloproteinase-12
- Microsomal epoxide hydrolase
- Glutathione S transferase
- Heme oxygenase 1
- Cytochrome P450 1A1
- Vitamin D binding protein

- Tumor necrosis factor α
- Interleukin-1
- Interleukin-1 receptor antagonist
- Interleukin-11
- Transforming growth factor $\beta1$
- Transforming growth factor β receptor 3
- Cystic fibrosis transmembrane regulator
- α_2-adrenergic receptor
- ABO-secretor status
- Microsatellite instability

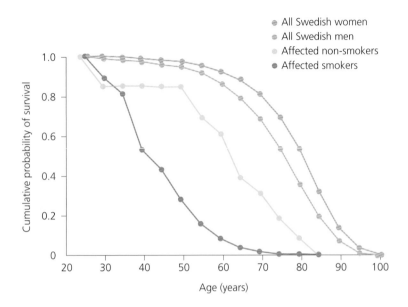

Figure 2.3 Cumulative probability of survival after 20 years of age for smoking and non-smoking individuals with α_1-proteinase inhibitor deficiency compared with the total population. Data from Larsson 1978.

these candidate genes can affect proteinase or oxidant balance, suggesting mechanisms of action analogous to those in α_1-proteinase inhibitor deficiency.

Inhibition of tissue repair may contribute to the development of COPD alongside the mechanisms that augment tissue destruction. Starvation, for example, has been reported to cause COPD both in humans and in animals. Moreover, starvation can exacerbate proteinase-induced emphysema in animal models. Such a mechanism may have clinical relevance. Many individuals with seemingly stable COPD often deteriorate if they develop a severe and prolonged intercurrent illness. Thus one of the benefits of careful attention to nutritional balance in such patients might be mitigation of the acceleration of COPD.

Other factors can also contribute. For example, emphysema has been reported in patients with human immunodeficiency virus (HIV) infection. In this context, the inflammation associated with HIV may be a contributing factor independent of cigarette smoke.

Progression of clinical symptoms

Current understanding of the natural history of COPD depends on assessment of FEV_1. Nevertheless, other clinical disease parameters, independent of FEV_1, are important. Weight loss, for example, is a bad prognostic sign; survival in COPD patients is negatively correlated with body mass index (Figure 2.4). Similarly, measures of health status (or 'quality of life') correlate significantly, but weakly, with FEV_1. Other factors such as exacerbations seem to be more important in driving health status, particularly in severely affected individuals.

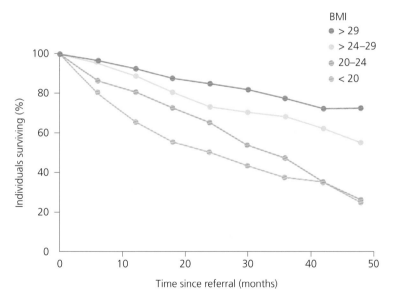

Figure 2.4 Weight as a prognostic sign in COPD: survival is negatively correlated with body mass index. The data represent 400 consecutive COPD patients referred for rehabilitation, who received no special dietary intervention. BMI, body mass index (mass [kg]/height^2 [m^2]). Data from Schols AM, Slangen J, Volovics L, Wouters EF. Weight loss is a reversible factor in the prognosis of chronic obstructive pulmonary disease. *Am J Respir Crit Care Med* 1998;157:1791–7.

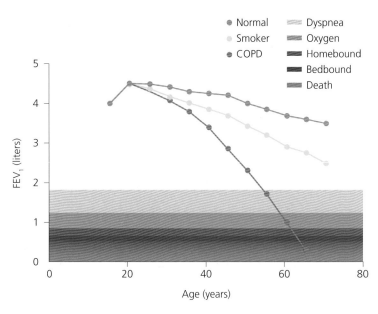

Figure 2.5 The natural history of COPD. The clinical features are related to averages for forced expiratory volume in 1 second (FEV_1); there are marked individual variations. Data adapted from Fletcher et al. 1976, 1977.

It is important, therefore, to view the natural history of COPD not only in terms of the decline in FEV_1, but also in terms of increasing symptoms. Figure 2.5 indicates the times of onset of symptoms, but these are averages. Many individuals will have symptoms at a much earlier stage, and some will progress to very limited airflow without being symptomatic. Some of the variation in symptomatic natural history is probably due to the fact that dyspnea is not directly related to FEV_1. Rather, with exertion, tachypnea ensues. This can lead to dynamic hyperinflation, and it is the increase in inspiratory work that is generally perceived as dyspnea. Many people who are developing COPD control dyspnea on exertion by decreasing their level of effort. As a result, they forgo activities as their disease progresses. Often this is attributed to aging or is accepted as 'normal' in a smoker, and subjects can become severely limited before presenting with symptoms.

The fact that individuals with COPD can be compromised at early stages of the disease without complaining of symptoms is a major reason for encouraging early diagnosis. Initiation of appropriate therapy early may improve patient function and quality of life, while preventing the severe deconditioning that routinely accompanies progressive COPD. Early recognition and intervention is a major goal of the new Global initiative for chronic Obstructive Lung Disease (GOLD) classification, and contrasts with older staging systems, in which a greater emphasis was placed on end-stage disease.

Key points – etiology and natural history

- Cigarette smoking is the most important risk factor for COPD; about 80% of COPD patients are, or have been, smokers.
- Almost all smokers develop impaired lung function. A diagnosis of COPD is made in about 15% of smokers, as many do not seek help for their functional compromise.
- Other influences, including air pollution and occupational exposures, contribute to COPD risk.
- Individual genetic susceptibility probably accounts for the heterogeneity of COPD risk.
- It is likely that many specific genetic factors will contribute to COPD risk, though only one, α_1-proteinase inhibitor deficiency, has been unequivocally identified.
- Asthma may contribute to COPD risk in some individuals.
- Early life events, including compromised lung development and growth, are likely to contribute to the risk of developing COPD later.

Key references

Barker DJ, Godfrey KM, Fall C et al. Relation of birth weight and childhood respiratory infection to adult lung function and death from chronic obstructive airways disease. BMJ 1991;303:671–5.

Burrows B, Knudson RJ, Cline MG et al. Quantitative relationships between cigarette smoking and ventilatory function. Am Rev Respir Dis 1979;115:751–60.

Fletcher C, Peto R. The natural history of chronic airflow obstruction. *BMJ* 1977;1:1645–8.

Fletcher C, Peto R, Tinker C, Speizer FE. *The Natural History of Chronic Bronchitis and Emphysema: An Eight-Year Study of Early Chronic Obstructive Lung Disease in Working Men in London.* New York: Oxford University Press, 1976:1–272.

Larsson C. Natural history and life expectancy in severe α_1-antitrypsin deficiency, Pi Z. *Acta Med Scand* 1978;204:345–51.

O'Donnell DE, Lam M, Webb KA. Measurement of symptoms, lung hyperinflation, and endurance during exercise in chronic obstructive pulmonary disease. *Am J Respir Crit Care Med* 1998;158:1557–65.

Postma DS, Boezen HM. The natural history of chronic obstructive pulmonary disease. *Eur Respir Mon* 2006;38:71–83.

Sandford AJ, Joos L, Paré PD. Genetic risk factors for chronic obstructive pulmonary disease. *Curr Opin Pulm Med* 2002;8:87–94.

Schols AM, Mostert R, Soeters PB, Wouters EF. Body composition and exercise performance in patients with chronic obstructive pulmonary disease. *Thorax* 1991;46:695–9.

Shapiro SD, Snider GL, Rennard SI. Chronic bronchitis and emphysema. In: Mason RJ, Broadus VC, Murray JF, Nadel JA, eds. *Textbook of Respiratory Medicine, 4th edn.* Philadelphia: WB Saunders, 2005:1115–67.

Symptoms

The characteristic symptom of COPD is breathlessness on exertion, sometimes accompanied by wheeze and cough, which is often, but not invariably, productive. Breathlessness is the symptom that commonly causes the patient to seek medical attention, and it is usually the most disabling of these symptoms. Patients often date the onset of their illness from an episode of worsening cough with sputum production, which leaves them with a degree of chronic breathlessness. However, close questioning will often reveal the presence of a 'smoker's cough' over a period of years, along with the production of small amounts (usually < 60 mL/day) of mucoid sputum, usually predominantly in the morning.

Most patients (80%) with COPD will have a smoking history of at least 20 pack-years (1 pack-year is equivalent to smoking 20 cigarettes, which is 1 pack, per day for 1 year or 10 a day for 2 years) before symptoms are recognized, commonly in the fifth decade. It is characteristic of patients with COPD to progress through the clinical stages of mild, moderate and severe disease. Symptoms and signs therefore vary in any individual depending on the stage of the disease. Considerable loss of lung function can occur before symptoms become apparent, and many patients may seek medical attention when the disease is at an advanced stage, since COPD is a slowly progressive disorder and patients gradually adapt their lives to their disability. Most smokers expect to cough and be short of breath, so they often dismiss these symptoms of progressive airflow limitation as a normal consequence of their smoking habit and the aging process.

Breathlessness is the symptom that causes most disability and is associated with loss of lung function over time. In good health, the body meets the increased oxygen demand produced by exercise by using some of the inspiratory reserve volume of the lungs to increase tidal volume (Figure 3.1). In COPD, because the caliber of the airways is relatively fixed, the inspiratory reserve volume cannot be fully utilized.

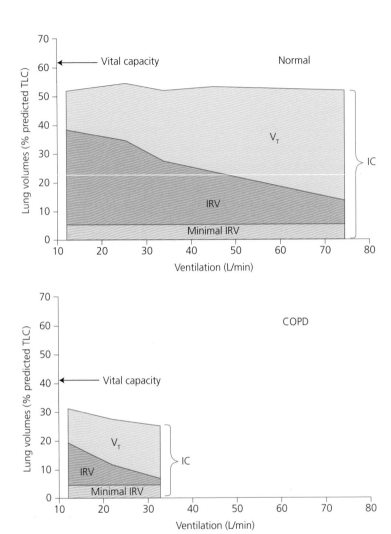

Figure 3.1 In good health, the body meets the increased oxygen demand of exercise by using some of the inspiratory reserve volume of the lungs to increase tidal volume. The presentation of the vertical axes are inverted from normal pulmonological convention for clarity. Data from O'Donnell DE, Revill SM, Webb KA. Dynamic hyperinflation and exercise intolerance in chronic obstructive pulmonary disease. *Am J Resp Crit Care Med* 2001;164:770–7. IC, inspiratory capacity; IRV, inspiratory reserve volume; TLC, total lung capacity; V_T, tidal volume.

Overinflation of the lungs with air trapped in the alveoli, particularly when the respiratory rate is increased, leads to increased residual volume at the expense of the inspiratory reserve volume, which worsens breathlessness. Airway collapse resulting from loss of alveolar support due to emphysema and consequent loss of the elastic recoil of the lungs causes more air trapping, further increasing the residual volume and increasing breathlessness on exertion. As the diaphragm flattens when the lungs are overinflated, the accessory muscles of respiration become increasingly important. The loss of alveolar/capillary surface in COPD, particularly in emphysema, means that the increased demand for oxygen imposed by exercise cannot be met, and this further increases the sensation of breathlessness.

In contrast to the variable breathlessness in asthma, the breathlessness in COPD is nearly constant, though some patients do report variation, particularly that breathlessness is worse in the morning.

Breathlessness is usually first noted while climbing hills or stairs, carrying heavy loads or hurrying on level ground. The appearance of breathlessness heralds moderate-to-severe airflow limitation. By the time the patient seeks medical advice, the forced expiratory volume in 1 second (FEV_1) has usually fallen to around 1–1.5 liters in an average man (30–45% of the expected value). Patients with COPD may adapt their breathing pattern and their behavior to minimize the sensation of breathlessness. Generally, this takes the form of greatly restricted activity.

The perception of breathlessness varies greatly between individuals with the same degree of ventilatory capacity. Breathlessness can be assessed using the modified Borg Scale (Table 3.1), a visual analog scale or the Medical Research Council (MRC) Dyspnea Scale (Table 3.2). Mood is an important determinant of the perception of breathlessness in patients with COPD. When the FEV_1 has fallen to 30% or less of the predicted value (equivalent in an average man to an FEV_1 of around 1 liter), breathlessness is usually present on minimal exertion. Severe breathlessness is often affected by changes in temperature and by exposure to dust and fumes. Position has a variable effect on breathlessness. Some patients have severe orthopnea, relieved by leaning forward, whereas others find the greatest ease when lying flat.

TABLE 3.1

The modified Borg scale for assessing breathlessness

Scale	Severity experienced by patient
0	Nothing at all
0.5	Very, very slight (just noticeable)
1	Very slight
2	Slight (light)
3	Moderate
4	Somewhat severe
5	Severe (heavy)
6	
7	Very severe
8	
9	Very, very severe (almost maximal)
10	Maximal

Cough and sputum production. A productive cough occurs in up to 50% of cigarette smokers. It may either precede or appear simultaneously with the onset of breathlessness, and occurs in association with breathlessness in 75% of patients with COPD. The MRC symptom questionnaire, which is used in epidemiological studies, employs cough as a defining symptom of chronic bronchitis, meaning a cough that produces sputum on most days for 3 consecutive months, over 2 consecutive years. Cessation of cigarette smoking produces resolution of the cough in over 90% of smokers; however, the airflow limitation often persists. Cough is often worse in the morning and, in contrast to asthma, nocturnal cough does not appear to be increased in stable COPD. In the presence of severe airway obstruction, the generation of high intrathoracic pressures may produce syncope during paroxysms of cough and 'cough fractures' of the ribs. Cough may also be exacerbated by gastroesophageal reflux.

Sputum production is a common, though not universal, feature of COPD. Sputum is usually white or gray in color, but may become

TABLE 3.2

The modified Medical Research Council dyspnea scale for assessing breathlessness

Grade	Degree of breathlessness related to activities
1	Not troubled by breathlessness except on strenuous exercise
2	Short of breath when hurrying or walking up a slight hill
3	Walks slower than contemporaries on the level because of breathlessness, or has to stop for breath when walking at own pace
4	Stops for breath after walking about 100 m or after a few minutes on the level
5	Too breathless to leave the house, or breathless when dressing or undressing

mucopurulent and green or yellow in color during exacerbations. However, some patients with COPD have persistently purulent sputum; this may relate to bacterial colonization in the airway. Indeed, it is now recognized that a number of such patients have underlying bronchiectasis. Excessive sputum production (more than 60 mL/day) should raise the possibility of bronchiectasis.

Hemoptysis can occur in exacerbations of COPD in association with infection, but should always be treated seriously, since the incidence of bronchial carcinoma is high in patients with COPD. The production of copious amounts of frothy sputum, particularly in association with orthopnea or hypertension and/or ischemic heart disease, raises the possibility of left ventricular failure and pulmonary edema.

Wheeze is common in COPD, but is not universally present and is a non-specific symptom. It is not easy to evaluate because of its intermittent nature and the difficulties patients experience in understanding this symptom. Wheeze is due to turbulent airflow through the larger airways as a result of various causes including bronchial smooth muscle contraction, structural airway narrowing and the presence of excess airway secretions. Wheeze does not usually wake patients with COPD at night as it does those with asthma. The absence of signs of wheeze on auscultation of the chest does not exclude a diagnosis of COPD.

Other symptoms. Chest pain is common in patients with COPD, but is often unrelated to the disease itself, and may be due to underlying ischemic heart disease or gastroesophageal reflux. Patients with COPD often complain of chest tightness during exacerbations of breathlessness, particularly during exercise, and this is sometimes difficult to distinguish from ischemic cardiac pain. Pleuritic chest pain may suggest an intercurrent pneumothorax, pneumonia or pulmonary infarction.

Weight loss is a feature of severe COPD and is thought to result from anorexia, decreased calorie intake and increased metabolism.

Psychiatric morbidity, particularly depression, is common in patients with severe COPD, which is likely to reflect the social isolation and the chronicity of the disease. Sleep quality is impaired in advanced COPD, which may contribute to the impaired neuropsychiatric performance.

History

A detailed history is important in COPD and should include:

- full smoking history
- exposure to other risk factors, particularly gases or dusts, and an occupational history
- medical history including asthma, allergy, sinusitis, nasal polyps, respiratory infection in childhood and other respiratory diseases
- family history of COPD or other chronic respiratory disease
- symptom development
- exacerbations or previous hospitalizations for respiratory disorders
- presence of comorbidity such as heart disease that may also contribute to the restriction of activity
- appropriateness of current medical treatment
- impact of the disease on the patient's life, including limitation of activity, work days lost and economic impact, effect on family and feelings of depression or anxiety
- social and family support available to the patient.

COPD is relatively uncommon among non-smokers and thus details of the patient's exposure to cigarettes, measured in pack-years, is important. Usually, symptomatic COPD develops after 20 pack-years of smoking (see page 31 for definition of pack-year). Most patients with COPD are over the age of 40. Similar signs in younger patients with much briefer smoking histories should raise suspicion of another condition and lead to a review of the other possible diagnoses or increased genetic susceptibility to COPD, such as α_1-antitrypsin deficiency. There is, in general, a dose-response relationship between the number of cigarettes smoked and the FEV_1; however, there are huge individual variations (see Figure 2.1, page 21), reflecting the varying susceptibility to cigarette smoke.

Occupational exposure to dusts has an additive effect on the decline in lung function, which has particularly been shown in coal miners, in whom both smoking and years of dust exposure contribute to the decline in FEV_1. Similar additive effects have been observed with air pollution. The contribution of smoking, however, is three times as great as that of dust exposure in miners.

Physical signs

The physical signs seen in patients with COPD are not specific to the disease. They depend on the degree of airflow limitation and pulmonary overinflation, and may be virtually absent in patients with mild-to-moderate disease, so their sensitivity in detecting or excluding COPD is poor. Physical signs of airflow limitation are rarely present until lung function is significantly impaired. Detection of early COPD is possible only by spirometry or by imaging techniques, such as high-resolution computed tomography (HRCT) to detect emphysema.

Breathing pattern. Patients with COPD often have a characteristic breathing pattern with a prolonged expiratory phase. Some patients adopt purse-lipped breathing on expiration, which may reduce expiratory airway collapse. The use of the accessory muscles of respiration, particularly the sternomastoids, is often seen in advanced disease; these patients often lean forward, supporting themselves with

37

their arms to fix the shoulder girdle, thus allowing the use of the pectorals and the latissimus dorsi to increase chest wall movement.

Signs of overinflation may be present. These are:

- increased anterior/posterior diameter of the chest, which when greater than the lateral diameter is described as a 'barrel-shaped chest'
- horizontal ribs with prominent sternal angle and wide subcostal angle
- reduced distance between the suprasternal notch and the cricoid cartilage (normally three finger-breadths)
- inspiratory tracheal tug
- Hoover's sign, which is when the horizontal position of the diaphragm acts to pull in the lower ribs during inspiration
- increased intrathoracic pressure swings may result in indrawing of the suprasternal and supraclavicular fossae and the intercostal muscles
- percussion of the chest may show decreased hepatic and cardiac dullness, indicating overinflation; a useful sign of gross overinflation is the absence of a dull percussion note, normally due to the underlying heart, over the lower end of the sternum.

Breath sounds may have a prolonged expiratory phase, or may be uniformly diminished, particularly in the advanced stages of the disease. Wheeze may be heard by the unaided ear, at the patient's mouth if necessary, and may be variably present on auscultation both on inspiration and expiration. Crackles may be present, particularly at the lung bases, but are usually scanty, vary with coughing and cannot be distinguished from the coarse crackles of bronchiectasis or fine respiratory crackles of fibrosis or left ventricular failure.

Different degrees of tachypnea may be present in patients with severe COPD, and prolonged forced expiratory time (> 5 seconds) can be a useful indicator of airway obstruction.

Physical appearance. Tar-stained fingers are an indication of a smoking habit. In advanced disease, cyanosis may be present, indicating hypoxemia, but may be influenced by the background lighting or accentuated by polycythemia, and therefore is a fairly subjective sign. The flapping tremor associated with hypercapnia is neither sensitive nor specific, and the often reported papilledema associated with severe hypercapnia is in fact rarely seen.

Weight loss may be apparent in advanced disease, as well as a reduction in muscle mass.

Finger clubbing is not a manifestation of COPD and should suggest the possibility of complicating bronchial neoplasm, bronchiectasis or lung fibrosis.

Cardiovascular signs. Overinflation of the chest makes it difficult to locate the apex beat and reduces the cardiac dullness. The characteristic signs indicative of the presence or consequences of pulmonary arterial hypertension may be difficult to detect in advanced disease. The heave of right ventricular hypertrophy may be palpable at the lower left sternal edge or in the subcostal angle. Heart sounds are generally soft, though the second heart sound may be exaggerated in the second left intercostal space in the presence of pulmonary hypertension. Splitting of the second heart sound with an increased pulmonary component may be present. There may be a right-sided gallop rhythm, with a third sound audible in the fourth intercostal space to the left of the sternum or in the epigastrium.

The jugular venous pressure can be difficult to assess in patients with COPD as it varies widely with respiration and is difficult to discern because of the prominent accessory muscle activity. When the fluid retention of cor pulmonale occurs, there may be evidence of functional tricuspid incompetence, producing a pansystolic murmur at the left sternal edge.

Peripheral vasodilation accompanies hypercapnia, producing warm peripheries with a high-volume pulse. Pitting peripheral edema may be present as a result of fluid retention. However, other causes of edema, such as venous stasis, low serum albumin and deep venous thrombosis, should be considered.

Hepatic signs. The liver may be tender and pulsatile, and a prominent 'v' wave may be visible in the jugular venous pulse. The liver may also be palpable below the right costal margin as a result of the low diaphragm due to the overinflation of the lungs.

Clinical presentation

Many smokers accept the development of exertional dyspnea and cough with sputum production as an inevitable consequence of the smoking habit, and therefore often present to their doctor when the disease is at a fairly advanced stage. Relatively few patients are diagnosed early in the course of the disease. Repeated spirometry over the course of several years will identify smokers with a rapid decline in FEV_1, who could be targeted for smoking cessation and early therapeutic intervention.

Some patients present initially to hospital or to their primary care provider during an exacerbation of the disease and claim that they had no significant symptoms until that time. However, close questioning often reveals the presence of progressive symptoms.

Two clinical patterns have been described, which are now recognized to be at either end of a clinical spectrum – the so-called 'pink puffers' and 'blue bloaters'. The pink and puffing patient is thin and breathless, and has blood gas values that are preserved until late in the course of the disease, and therefore does not develop pulmonary hypertension until the disease is very advanced. By contrast, the blue and bloated patient develops hypoxemia and hypercapnia earlier, and thus also the complications of edema and secondary polycythemia. Most patients lie between these two extremes. These 'phenotypes' are not indicative of emphysema or bronchitis, as was once thought, but clearly indicate the varied systemic manifestations of COPD.

Systemic effects

Traditionally, COPD is regarded as a disease of the lungs characterized by progressive symptoms and a decline in lung function. Therapeutic strategies such as bronchodilators and inhaled glucocorticosteroids have therefore been used for relieving symptoms in association with improving airflow limitation. However, COPD is also associated with a number of systemic effects and comorbidities (Table 3.3)

Exercise limitation is a common complaint in COPD and is usually explained on the basis of the increased work of breathing caused by airflow limitation. However, almost 50% of patients with COPD stop exercising because of leg fatigue, not because of breathlessness. This

TABLE 3.3

Systemic effects and comorbidities in COPD

- Cardiac
  - Infarction
  - Arrhythmia
  - Heart failure
- Hypercoagulability
  - Stroke
  - Deep vein thrombosis
  - Pulmonary embolism
- Aortic aneurysm
- Osteoporosis
- Weight loss

- Skeletal muscle weakness
- Skin wrinkling
- Diabetes mellitus
- Glaucoma
- Peptic ulceration
- Gastroesophageal reflux
- Anemia
- Fluid retention
- Depression
- Lung cancer

suggests that skeletal muscle dysfunction is an important factor in the symptom complex. Skeletal muscle dysfunction is a good predictor of poor exercise performance, correlating more strongly than either lung function or blood gas measurements. This dysfunction is not entirely due to a sedentary lifestyle, but the mechanisms involved are not yet fully understood, though limited oxygen delivery or cellular changes in the skeletal muscle consequent on the inflammatory processes underlying COPD may be implicated.

Many COPD patients lose weight during the course of their disease (see Figure 2.4, page 27). This phenomenon is of prognostic value, and is independent of the more traditional prognostic factors related to FEV_1 and the partial pressure of oxygen in arterial blood (PaO_2). The mechanisms underlying the weight loss are unclear, but may be related to the increased metabolic rate, tissue hypoxia and systemic inflammation.

Osteoporosis is more common in COPD patients than in the general population. This may be due, in part, to concurrent smoking and to the use of corticosteroids. COPD itself, however, appears to be associated with bone mineral loss.

General population studies and studies in patients with COPD suggest that COPD is an important risk factor for ischemic heart disease and sudden cardiac death. Indeed, the FEV_1 is an established predictor of cardiovascular mortality. The mechanism responsible for the increased risk of cardiovascular disease in patients with COPD is unknown, but a number of hypotheses have been proposed including the effect of systemic inflammation and endothelial dysfunction.

COPD, in particular emphysema, also increases the risk of lung cancer. The mechanism is again unclear, but may result from common risk factors such as smoking, the involvement of susceptibility genes or failure to clear carcinogens.

COPD is characterized by an excessive inflammatory process in the lung parenchyma in response to inhaled particles or gases. Evidence of inflammation has also been detected in the systemic circulation, such as markers of oxidative stress, elevated levels of cytokines and activation of circulating leukocytes.

Key points – clinical features

- COPD is uncommon, but not unknown, in those who do not smoke.
- Usually (80% of patients) there is a significant smoking history of at least 20 pack-years. For those with lesser smoking histories or for younger individuals, consider an alternative diagnosis or a genetic predisposition (e.g. α_1-antitrypsin deficiency).
- The most common and most distressing symptom in COPD is breathlessness on exertion.
- Symptoms and signs often present only at an advanced stage of the disease.
- Clinical signs may not be apparent in mild disease. They include signs of overinflation, prominent use of accessory muscles of respiration, weight loss, expiratory wheeze, cyanosis, peripheral edema and raised jugular venous pressure.
- The systemic effects of COPD result in a number of comorbidities that impact on the morbidity and mortality of the disease.

Comorbid conditions (see Table 3.3) have an important effect on morbidity and mortality, and should be comprehensively assessed and managed in all COPD patients.

Spectrum of disease

Many national and international guidelines for COPD have used a simple classification of disease severity based on spirometry. The most recent classification from the Global initiative for chronic Obstructive Lung Disease (GOLD) also includes symptoms (see Table 4.1, page 48).

Key references

Agusti AGN. Systemic effects of COPD. *Proc Am Thorac Soc* 2007;4:522–5.

Calverley PM, Georgopoulos D. Chronic obstructive pulmonary disease: symptoms and signs. *Eur Respir Mon* 2006;38:7–23.

Fabbri LM, Luppi F, Beghé B, Rabe KF. Complex comorbidities of COPD. *Eur Respir J* 2008;31: 204–12.

MacNee W. Chronic bronchitis and emphysema. In: Seaton A, Seaton D, Leitch AG, eds. *Crofton and Douglas's Respiratory Diseases 1*. Oxford: Blackwell Science, 2000: 616–95.

Spirometry

The most important disturbance of respiratory function in COPD is obstruction to forced expiratory flow. The degree of airflow obstruction cannot be predicted from the symptoms and signs, and therefore assessment of the degree and the progression of airway obstruction should be encouraged in both primary and secondary care. To identify patients early in the course of the disease, spirometry should be performed for those who have chronic cough and sputum production, and for those at risk, such as smokers, even if they have no dyspnea. In the early stages of the disease, conventional spirometry may reveal no abnormality. This is because the earliest changes in COPD affect the alveolar walls and small airways. The resulting modest increase in peripheral airway resistance is not reflected in the conventional spirometric measurements. A reduction in forced expiratory volume in 1 second (FEV_1) relative to vital capacity may, however, be a more sensitive measure. Similarly, sequential measures, which track changes in lung function, may also be more sensitive indicators. Spirometry is the most robust test of airflow limitation in patients with COPD.

Spirometry assesses the volume of exhaled air over time and is performed with the patient exhaling from a maximum inhalation to a maximum exhalation using maximum force to blow out all the air as hard and as fast as possible. In healthy individuals, this forced expiratory maneuver can be completed in 3–4 seconds but, in patients with increasing airflow limitation, it may take up to 15 seconds. The volume of air exhaled is plotted on a graph against the time taken to reach the maximum exhalation (Figure 4.1). Three indices can then be derived:

- forced expiratory volume in 1 second (FEV_1)
- forced vital capacity (FVC), which is the total volume of air that can be exhaled from a maximum inhalation to a maximum exhalation
- the ratio of FEV_1 to FVC, expressed as a percentage.

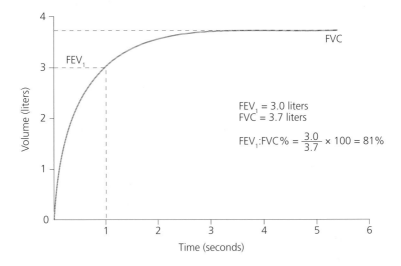

Figure 4.1 Normal spirometry. FEV$_1$, forced expiratory volume in 1 second; FVC, forced vital capacity.

FEV$_1$ and FVC are expressed in absolute values in liters and also as a percentage of the predicted values for the individual depending on their age, height, sex and ethnic origin. Values within ± 20% of the predicted values are considered to be within the normal range. Thus an FEV$_1$ of over 80% of the predicted value is considered to be normal. Under normal circumstances, 70–80% of the total volume of the air in the lungs (the FVC) should be exhaled in the first second. In other words, the FEV$_1$:FVC ratio is normally 70–80%. When airflow through the airways is obstructed, it is not possible to exhale so much air in the first second, and the FEV$_1$:FVC ratio falls. A ratio of less than 70% indicates airflow obstruction (Figure 4.2). A post-bronchodilator FEV$_1$:FVC ratio below the normal range indicates chronic airflow limitation and is a diagnostic criterion for COPD.

The use of a fixed FEV$_1$:FVC ratio as a diagnostic criterion for chronic airflow limitation is a pragmatic approach, as reference values for FEV$_1$:FVC are unavailable. The use of the fixed ratio is, however, problematic because the ratio declines with age with the potential for

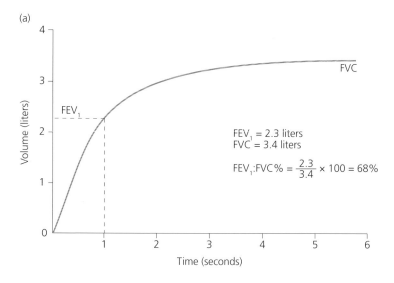

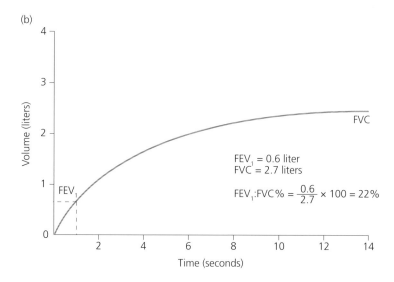

Figure 4.2 (a) Spirometry showing mild obstruction. (b) Spirometry showing severe obstruction. FEV_1, forced expiratory volume in 1 second; FVC, forced vital capacity.

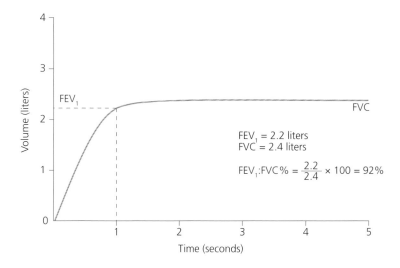

Figure 4.3 Spirometry showing a restrictive defect; the FEV_1:FVC ratio is within the normal range. FEV_1, forced expiratory volume in 1 second; FVC, forced vital capacity.

overdiagnosis of COPD in the elderly. Some guidelines suggest that an additional criterion for the diagnosis of COPD should be an FEV_1 of less than 80% of that predicted.

In airway obstruction, the FEV_1 is reduced both in terms of volume and as a percentage of the predicted value. The FVC also falls, but less than the FEV_1, so that the FEV_1:FVC ratio decreases (see Figure 4.2). By contrast, in restrictive defects, such as lung fibrosis or chest-wall deformity, the airway size remains normal, but both the FEV_1 and FVC are reduced, so the ratio remains above 70% (Figure 4.3).

Classification of severity. Patients with COPD typically show a decrease in both the FEV_1 and the FEV_1:FVC ratio (the latter being a more sensitive measure of early airflow limitation). The degree of spirometric abnormality generally reflects the severity of COPD and is used as part of the classification (Table 4.1). However, spirometry alone does not provide a complete assessment of severity, particularly with respect to functional status. In addition to spirometry, assessment

TABLE 4.1

GOLD classification of severity of COPD

Stage	Characteristics
I: mild COPD	• FEV_1:FVC < 70% • $FEV_1 \geq 80\%$ predicted • With or without chronic symptoms (cough, sputum production)
II: moderate COPD	• FEV_1:FVC < 70% • 50% ≤ FEV_1 < 80% predicted
III: severe COPD	• FEV_1:FVC < 70% • 30% ≤ FEV_1 < 50% predicted
IV: very severe COPD	• FEV_1:FVC < 70% • FEV_1 < 30% predicted or FEV_1 < 50% predicted plus chronic respiratory failure

FEV_1, post-bronchodilator forced expiratory volume in 1 second; FVC, forced vital capacity; GOLD, Global initiative for chronic Obstructive Lung Disease. Source: Global Initiative for Chronic Obstructive Lung Disease. *Global Strategy for the Diagnosis, Management, and Prevention of Chronic Obstructive Pulmonary Disease. NHLBI/WHO Workshop Report.* Updated 2008. www.goldcopd.com

of severity should include evaluation of symptoms, exercise capacity and the presence of systemic effects, comorbidities and complications, such as respiratory failure and right heart failure. One approach to assess severity that incorporates these variables is the BODE index (Body mass index, Obstruction, Dyspnea, Exercise; Table 4.2), which is a better predictor of mortality than any individual variable alone.

Technique. It is important that a volume plateau is reached in spirometry. This can take 15 seconds or more in a patient with severe airway obstruction. If this maneuver is not carried out properly, the FVC can be underestimated. Many spirometers currently in use substitute the forced expiratory volume in 6 seconds for FVC. Such instruments therefore underestimate the vital capacity, and thus yield artificially elevated FEV_1:FVC ratios. This limitation is not felt to be a major impediment for the diagnosis of COPD (the criterion being a ratio < 70%), but it does reduce the reliability of the ratio as a gauge of disease severity.

Since FEV_1 is effort-dependent, traces should be checked to ensure that maximum effort has been achieved and that full expiration has been performed. The FEV_1 is very reproducible and varies by less than 170 mL between maneuvers if the test is carried out correctly. The test reproducibility is an excellent measure of the effort exerted by the patient and the quality of the test. In contrast to maximal efforts, which are highly reproducible, submaximal efforts are highly variable. Therefore, reproducibility of the tests to within ± 2% is generally regarded as a measure of satisfactory test quality; many modern spirometers can perform such assessments automatically. The FVC also depends on effort, particularly during the latter part of the maneuver, and results are more variable. To avoid the effect of airway collapse in patients with COPD during a forced expiratory maneuver, it is suggested that a relaxed or slow vital capacity (VC) measurement, in which the patient exhales at his/her own pace after maximum

TABLE 4.2

Variables and point values used for the computation of the BODE index

Variable	Points on BODE index			
	0	1	2	3
FEV_1 (% of predicted)	≥ 65	50–64	36–49	≤ 35
Distance walked in 6 minutes (m)	≥ 350	250–349	150–249	≤ 149
MRC dyspnea scale*	0–1	2	3	4
Body mass index	> 21	≤ 21		

*See Table 3.2, page 35.
BODE, body mass index, degree of airflow obstruction and dyspnea, and exercise capacity; FEV_1, forced expiratory volume in 1 second; MRC, Medical Research Council.

inhalation, should be used. The slow VC is often 0.5 liters greater than the FVC. With increasing airflow obstruction, it takes longer to exhale and the early slope of the volume–time trace becomes less steep (see Figure 4.2b).

In assessing FEV_1, the following points should be remembered.

- Patients should be clinically stable (i.e. at least 4 weeks must have passed since the last exacerbation).
- If patients have taken a bronchodilator, results may be improved from 'baseline'.
- Patients should be sitting in an upright position.
- An adequate explanation of the technique should be given.
- Patients should be asked to take a maximum breath in and then place their lips around the mouthpiece, forming an airtight seal.
- Patients should then be encouraged to exhale as hard, as fast and as completely as possible.
- Adequate time should be allowed for recovery between exhalations, with a maximum of six forced maneuvers being performed in one session.
- Three technically satisfactory maneuvers giving similar results should be carried out.
- At least two readings of FEV_1 should be within 100 mL or 5% of each other.

Peak expiratory flow

Peak expiratory flow (PEF) can either be read directly from the flow–volume loop (see page 54) or measured with a handheld peak flowmeter. It is a simple, quick and inexpensive way of measuring airflow obstruction, and has been particularly useful for repeated measurements in patients with asthma to reveal spontaneous diurnal variation or variations in response to therapy. The PEF meter measures the maximal flow rate that can be maintained over 10 ms; it is most effective for monitoring changes in airflow in an individual over time, but has less value in diagnosis. In COPD, there is little daily change in PEF and many of the variations are often within the error range of the measurement. Although repeated measurements of PEF can replace measurement of FEV_1, single measurements are not useful as the variation is so high. There are several theoretical reasons why FEV_1 is a better measurement than PEF in the diagnosis and assessment of COPD (Table 4.3).

TABLE 4.3

Reasons why FEV_1 is the measurement of choice in COPD

- It is a reproducible and objective measurement. There are well-defined normal ranges that allow for the effects of age, race and sex
- It is relatively simple and quick to measure and can be measured at all stages of disease
- The forced expiratory maneuver records not only FEV_1, but also FVC. An FEV_1:FVC ratio < 70% is diagnostic of airway obstruction. If the ratio is normal (> 70%) and the test was performed well, the pattern is not obstructive and the diagnosis is not COPD
- PEF measurements cannot determine whether values are low because of obstruction or restriction
- The variance of repeated FEV_1 measurements in the same person is well documented and is low
- Studies of mortality and disability have shown that the FEV_1 predicts future mortality from COPD and other respiratory and cardiac diseases
- Serial measurements provide evidence of disease progression
- In COPD, the relationship between PEF and FEV_1 is poor
- PEF may underestimate the degree of airway obstruction in COPD
- FEV_1 is better related to prognosis and disability than FEV_1:FVC ratio, because the FVC depends on effort and is therefore more variable

FEV_1, forced expiratory volume in 1 second; FVC, forced vital capacity; PEF, peak expiratory flow.

Reversibility testing

Bronchodilators. The main objectives of a bronchodilator reversibility test in COPD are:

- to help distinguish those patients with marked reversibility who have underlying asthma (it is the post-bronchodilator lung function that defines the presence and severity of COPD)
- to establish the post-bronchodilator FEV_1, which is the best predictor of long-term prognosis
- to establish the best obtainable lung function.

There is no agreement on a standardized method of assessing reversibility. Usually changes in the FEV_1 or PEF are monitored, but reversibility could also be determined as a change in static lung volumes after administration of a bronchodilator.

The use of bronchodilator testing in patients with COPD is limited by the variability of the FEV_1 measurement itself, and by the fact that, by definition, patients with COPD may have only a small degree of reversibility, which is often within the error of the measurement. Bronchodilator reversibility tests can also vary from day to day depending on the degree of bronchomotor tone. A change in FEV_1 that exceeds 170 mL can be considered not to have occurred by chance. Most guidelines recommend that changes should be considered significant only if they exceed 200 mL. In addition to this absolute change in FEV_1, a percentage change of 12% over baseline has been suggested as significant by the American Thoracic Society and the Global initiative for chronic Obstructive Lung Disease guidelines, whereas an improvement of 15% over baseline FEV_1 and a 200 mL absolute change has been suggested by European Respiratory Society and British Thoracic Society guidelines.

Another approach to measuring reversibility is to express the change in FEV_1 as a percentage of the maximum potential change, which is the predicted value minus the baseline value.

Reversibility testing with a bronchodilator is generally indicated only at the time of diagnosis. Bronchodilator testing should usually be undertaken only in patients with COPD at stage II (moderate) and above, and reversibility testing should be conducted during a period of clinical stability, with a high dose of bronchodilator in order not to miss a significant response. The high dose can be delivered by means of a nebulizer. An alternative method is to deliver a smaller dose of the drug by giving repeated doses from a metered-dose inhaler through a large-volume spacer. The usual recommended protocol for testing bronchial reversibility is shown in Table 4.4. Improvement of lung function to normal suggests a diagnosis of asthma without the presence of COPD.

Daily variations in airway smooth muscle tone may affect the response to bronchodilators in patients with COPD. Thus when airway smooth muscle tone is higher and FEV_1 is therefore lower, a response to bronchodilators may be more likely than when muscle tone is lower and FEV_1 higher. One-third of those patients who are initially shown to have a response to a bronchodilator may, on retesting on a different day, have no response. Conversely, patients who do not show a significant FEV_1 response to a bronchodilator can still benefit symptomatically from long-term bronchodilator treatment.

TABLE 4.4

Guidelines for bronchodilator reversibility testing

- Withhold all bronchodilators for sufficient time for therapeutic effect to abate

- Record FEV_1 before and 15 minutes after giving salbutamol (albuterol)*, 2.5–5 mg, or nebulized terbutaline, 5–10 mg

- Record (preferably on a separate occasion) FEV_1 before and 30 minutes after nebulized ipratropium bromide, 500 μg

- Record (on a separate occasion) FEV_1 before and 30 minutes after a combination of salbutamol (albuterol) or terbutaline and ipratropium

*Salbutamol is the recommended international non-proprietary name favored by the World Health Organization, albuterol is the official generic name in the USA.
FEV_1, forced expiratory volume in 1 second.

Glucocorticosteroids. Reversibility after administration of corticosteroids is observed in 10–20% of patients with clinically stable COPD. Whether all patients with symptomatic COPD should undergo formal assessment of corticosteroid reversibility remains controversial. Those patients who have previously had a response to nebulized bronchodilators are more likely to respond to corticosteroids. However, it is not possible to predict the response to corticosteroids in any individual patient. Corticosteroid reversibility tests are usually performed during a period of clinical stability. Systemic corticosteroid challenge testing is not recommended. A 6-week or 3-month trial of inhaled corticosteroids, such as beclometasone (beclomethasone), 1000 µg/day, or its equivalent can be performed, but withdrawal may be associated with an exacerbation.

The criteria for a positive response are the same as in bronchodilator reversibility testing: a 200 mL and 15% improvement in the FEV_1 over baseline. Another criterion is an improvement of 20% or more in the mean PEF over the first 5 days and the last 5 days of a treatment trial. The response to corticosteroids is best evaluated with respect to the post-bronchodilator FEV_1; that is, the post-bronchodilator FEV_1 is measured, followed by measurement of any further improvement achieved with a corticosteroid, since the post-bronchodilator FEV_1 is the most reliable and least variable measurement from day to day. Improvements in symptoms or exercise tolerance following corticosteroids may be seen in those who show no significant FEV_1 response.

Neither bronchodilator nor oral corticosteroid reversibility testing or the small changes in FEV_1 (e.g. < 400 mL) that occur in COPD patients are predictive of disease progression or response to treatment. However, larger changes (> 400 mL) are suggestive of asthma.

Specialized lung function tests

Flow–volume loops. Many spirometers plot expiratory flow rate throughout the entire expiration at the same time as a standard volume–time trace. The PEF, which is sustained for 10 ms, represents the flow only in the larger airways. However, the flow–volume trace interprets flow from all generations of the airways and may be more helpful than PEF in detecting early airway narrowing in smaller airways

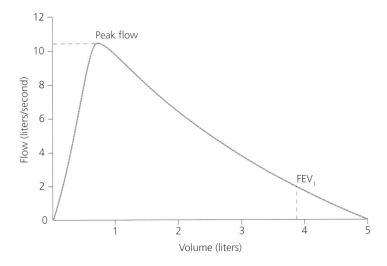

Figure 4.4 Normal flow–volume curve.

(Figure 4.4). Expiratory flow rates at 75% or 50% of VC have been used as a measure of airflow limitation, and provide complementary information to that obtained from the usual volume–time plot. There are problems with the reproducibility of these measurements, so that values must fall below 50% of the predicted values to be considered abnormal. Flows at lung volumes below 50% of VC were previously considered to be an indicator of small-airways dysfunction, but probably provide no more clinically useful information than measurement of FEV_1. Examples of flow–volume loops in airflow obstruction are shown in Figure 4.5.

The flow–volume loop can also help to identify the presence of obstruction of the large airways. The patterns of obstruction can vary with inspiration and expiration.

Lung volumes. Measurements of static lung volumes, such as total lung capacity, residual volume and functional residual capacity (Figure 4.6), can be made using a body plethysmograph or the helium dilution technique. These measurements are used to assess the degree of overinflation and gas trapping resulting from loss of elastic recoil and collapse of the airways. It is known that dynamic overinflation occurs

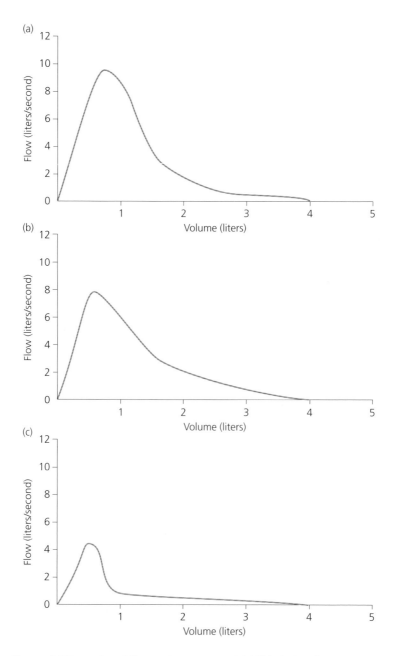

Figure 4.5 Examples of flow–volume curves. (a) Mild obstruction.
(b) Moderate obstruction. (c) Severe obstruction.

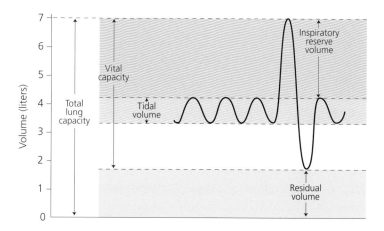

Figure 4.6 Lung volume measurements.

in COPD, particularly during exercise, and it may be an important determinant of symptoms such as breathlessness. Inspiratory capacity may be a useful surrogate for more precise measures of dynamic hyperinflation (see Figure 3.1, page 32).

The standard method for measuring static lung volumes using the helium dilution technique during rebreathing may underestimate lung volumes, particularly in patients with bullous disease, where the inspired helium does not have time to equilibrate properly in the airspaces. The body plethysmograph uses Boyle's law to calculate lung volumes from measurements of changes in mouth and body plethysmograph pressures during gentle panting against a closed shutter. This technique measures trapped air within the thorax and thus includes poorly ventilated areas, which therefore gives higher measurements than the helium dilution technique in COPD. Computed tomography (CT) scans on inhalation/exhalation can also be used to measure lung volumes.

Gas transfer by the lungs can be measured using carbon monoxide as a tracer gas. Following inhalation of a small amount of carbon monoxide, some of the inhaled marker is transferred from the lungs into the pulmonary capillary blood where it binds to hemoglobin. Reductions in the concentration of carbon monoxide in the exhaled gas

57

can therefore be used to gauge the efficiency of gas transfer within the lung. Some of the reduction in carbon monoxide level is also due to diffusion into the residual volume of the lung. Thus values for the diffusing capacity in the lung for carbon monoxide (DLco; TLco in the UK) are generally corrected using helium, which diffuses into the residual volume but is not absorbed into the pulmonary capillary blood. This technique yields the ventilated alveolar volume (V_A), which provides the carbon monoxide transfer coefficient Kco ($DLco/V_A$).

DLco values are normal in asthma, but below normal in many patients with COPD. Although there is a relationship between the DLco and the extent of emphysema, the severity of the emphysema in an individual patient cannot be predicted from the DLco. Neither is a low DLco specific for emphysema, as it can be affected by cigarette smoking, anemia and lung diseases, such as pulmonary fibrosis and pulmonary thromboembolism. Thus a low DLco in a patient with COPD suggests a significant degree of alveolar destruction, probably as a result of emphysema, but a normal DLco does not exclude a diagnosis of COPD. The principal factors affecting the DLco are:
- the thickness of the alveolar membrane
- capillary blood volume
- hemoglobin concentration (the test needs to be corrected for hemoglobin concentration).

The most widely used method for measuring DLco is the single-breath technique, which measures the rate of carbon monoxide uptake during a 10-second breath hold and uses alveolar volume calculated from helium dilution during the single-breath test. This will underestimate alveolar volume in patients with severe COPD.

Arterial blood gases and oximetry. In advanced COPD, measurement of arterial blood gases is important to assess the degree of hypoxemia and hypercapnia and, particularly in exacerbations, to define the partial pressure of carbon dioxide in arterial blood ($PaCO_2$) and the pH.

Arterial blood gases should be measured in patients with an FEV_1 of less than 50% of the predicted value, or when clinical signs suggest respiratory failure, right heart failure or cor pulmonale. Recording the inspired oxygen concentration is essential when reporting blood gases, but it is also important to note that it may take at least 30 minutes for a change in inspired oxygen concentration to have a full effect on the partial pressure of oxygen in arterial blood (PaO_2), because equilibration of alveolar gas takes a long time in COPD.

Blood for measurement of blood gases should be obtained by arterial puncture. Respiratory failure is indicated by a PaO_2 below 8 kPa (60 mmHg) with or without a $PaCO_2$ above 6.7 kPa (50 mmHg) while breathing air. Finger or ear oximeters for assessing oxygenation (percentage oxygen saturation of arterial blood, SaO_2) are less reliable but, because of their ease of use, are commonly used in clinical practice. An SaO_2 of 88% or below indicates the need for supplemental oxygen. Oximeters can also be used to measure changes in oxygenation during acute exacerbations. However, oximeters cannot completely replace assessment of blood gas values, because measurements of $PaCO_2$ are often required.

Increases in $PaCO_2$ can be compensated for by renal conservation of bicarbonate, which is a relatively slow process. Acid–base status, particularly in mixed respiratory and metabolic disturbances, can be characterized by plotting values on an acid–base diagram (Figure 4.7). It can also be assessed from the arterial pH and bicarbonate.

Exercise tests. Exercise induces an increase in oxygen consumption and carbon dioxide production in skeletal muscle. Patients with COPD have the same oxygen consumption for a given workload as normal individuals. However, their dead-space ventilation is higher and so a larger minute ventilation is needed to maintain carbon dioxide at a constant level. In many patients with COPD, expiratory airflow is limited within the tidal volume range. The only way to increase minute ventilation is to increase inspiratory flow or shift the end-expiratory position. Both of these maneuvers are problematic in patients with COPD and require more work from already compromised inspiratory muscles, or result in progressive overinflation, which increases both the work of breathing and symptoms.

In addition, the increased cardiac output that occurs with exercise can lead to increased perfusion of poorly ventilated areas. As a result of

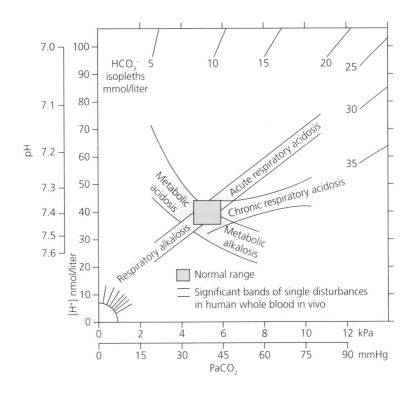

Figure 4.7 A non-logarithmic acid–base diagram derived from the measured acid–base status of patients within the five abnormal bands illustrated and of normal subjects (blue box). This plot of PaCO$_2$ against pH allows the likely acid–base disturbance and calculated bicarbonate value (obtained from the relevant isopleth) to be rapidly determined. Changes during treatment can be plotted serially for each patient. Reprinted from *The Lancet*. Flenley DC. Another non-logarithmic acid–base diagram? *Lancet* 1971;1:961–5, © 1971 with permission from Elsevier. HCO$_3$-, bicarbonate; PaCO$_2$, partial pressure of carbon dioxide in arterial blood.

this ventilation–perfusion mismatch, arterial oxygenation can decline with exercise in contrast to the improvement in oxygenation that is noted in normal individuals. Decline in oxygenation with exercise is generally monitored by measurement of percutaneous oxygen saturation. Exercise-induced desaturation can be an indication for supplemental oxygen therapy.

Three principal forms of exercise test are performed in COPD: progressive symptom-limited exercise, self-paced exercise and steady-state exercise. Other tests may be used in special circumstances.

Progressive symptom-limited exercise tests require patients to maintain exercise on a treadmill or a cycle until symptoms prevent them from continuing. The usual criteria for defining a maximum test are a heart rate greater than 85% of the predicted value or a ventilation greater than 90% of the predicted value. The results of the test are useful, particularly when simultaneous electrocardiography (ECG) and blood pressure monitoring are performed to assess whether coexisting cardiac or psychological factors contribute to exercise limitation.

Self-paced exercise tests are easy to perform and give information on more sustained exercise, which may be more relevant to performance in daily life. The 6-minute walk is the most commonly used test, with a coefficient of variation of around 8%. There may, however, be a learning effect that influences the result of repeated tests. This test is only useful in patients with moderately severe COPD ($FEV_1 < 1.5$ liters) who would be expected to have an exercise tolerance of less than 600 meters in 6 minutes. There is only a weak relationship between walking distance and FEV_1. The shuttle walking test is an alternative in which the patient performs a paced walk between two points 10 meters apart (a shuttle). The pace of the walk is increased at regular intervals, dictated by bleeps on a tape recording, until the patient is forced to stop because of breathlessness. The number of completed shuttles is recorded.

Steady-state exercise tests require exercise at a sustainable percentage of maximum capacity for 3–6 minutes while blood gases are measured, enabling calculation of the dead space:tidal volume ratio and the passage through the lungs without oxygenation (shunt). This assessment is seldom required in patients with COPD.

Other more complex tests, such as assessing the lung pressure–volume curve, are difficult to undertake, because they require measurement of esophageal pressure with an esophageal balloon, and are not part of the routine assessment, but may be necessary in special circumstances. Measurements of small airway function, such as the nitrogen washout test, helium and air flow–volume loops and frequency dependency of compliance (the dependence of lung compliance on respiratory frequency), have poor reproducibility in patients with COPD. Although they can differentiate smokers from non-smokers, they are not useful in predicting which smokers will develop COPD and thus are not used in routine practice.

Additional pulmonary function tests, such as inspiratory capacity and lung volumes, are not usually required in routine assessment, but can provide further information. They are useful in some cases in which the diagnosis is uncertain and in assessing patients for surgery.

Assessment of breathlessness

Improvement in symptoms, particularly breathlessness, is one of the important goals of treatment in COPD. Although breathlessness is a subjective feature, it should be quantified. Several scales are available for assessing breathlessness objectively (see Chapter 3).

The Medical Research Council (MRC) dyspnea scale (see Table 3.2, page 35) allows patients to rate their breathlessness according to the activity that induces it. It is graded from 0 to 5 and is easy to use, but it is insensitive to change and may be more valuable as a baseline assessment than as a means of measuring the effect of treatment.

The oxygen-cost diagram is more sensitive to change than the MRC dyspnea scale. It allows the patient to place a mark on a 10-cm line to represent the point beyond which breathlessness occurs (Figure 4.8). Other scales allow quantification of breathlessness according to the intensity of the sensation. The Borg scale (see Table 3.1, page 34) is useful for measuring short-term changes in the intensity of breathlessness during a particular task. It is sensitive and reproducible. A simple analog scale is another method of allowing patients to rate the intensity of their breathlessness. As with the oxygen-cost diagram, a 10-cm line is drawn on a page and the patient then marks on the line how intense their breathlessness is, from 'not at all' (0 cm) to 'intensely breathless' (10 cm). The score is the distance along the line that the patient has marked.

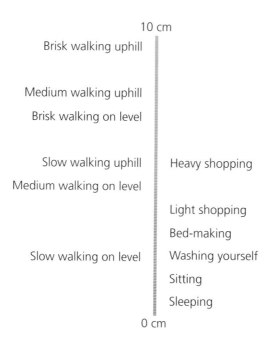

Figure 4.8 Oxygen-cost diagram used in the assessment of breathlessness. The patient places a mark on the line to indicate when breathlessness occurs. The distance in centimeters from the zero point can be used to obtain a score.

Health status

Health status, sometimes termed quality of life, is a measure of the impact of a disease on daily life and well-being. COPD has a marked effect on health status, particularly owing to the limitations posed by breathlessness on exercise, daily activities and social activities, as well as the reductions in expectations, mood and well-being that it causes. Several questionnaires are available for the measurement of health status, but they are mainly used in hospital rehabilitation programs and in research, and are not yet employed in clinical practice.

The Chronic Respiratory Disease Index Questionnaire is sensitive to change, but is very time-consuming and requires training to administer properly. The St George's Respiratory Questionnaire (SGRQ) is a self-completed questionnaire with three components that give a total score of overall health status: symptoms, measuring distress due to respiratory symptoms; activity, measuring disturbance of daily activities; and impact, measuring psychosocial function. The Breathing Problems Questionnaire is a similar self-completed questionnaire, which is easy to complete, but relatively insensitive to change. The SGRQ has been most validated in COPD. Although there is a relationship between the SGRQ and the FEV_1 as a percentage of the predicted value, the relationship is rather poor. It is clear from various studies that treatment-related improvement in the SGRQ health status can occur without any improvement in FEV_1. The threshold of clinical improvement is a change of four units in the SGRQ.

Exacerbations of COPD have a clear detrimental effect on health status.

Respiratory muscle function

Respiratory muscle function can be assessed by measuring maximum inspiratory and expiratory mouth pressure. These measurements can be useful in evaluating patients with breathlessness or exercise intolerance that is unexplained by the severity of the lung function abnormality, as well as patients with suspected peripheral muscle weakness.

Sleep studies

Patients with COPD become increasingly hypoxemic during sleep, particularly during rapid eye movement sleep. There is no evidence that measurement of nocturnal hypoxemia provides any further prognostic or clinically useful information in the assessment of patients with COPD unless coexisting sleep apnea syndrome is suspected. Individuals who desaturate during the night may, however, be candidates for oxygen therapy.

Other assessments

Polycythemia. In patients with severe COPD, identifying polycythemia is important since it predisposes to vascular events. Polycythemia should be suspected when the hematocrit is more than 47% in women and more than 52% in men, and/or the hemoglobin is greater than 16 g/dL in women and greater than 18 g/dL in men, provided other causes of spurious polycythemia due to decreased plasma volume, such as occurs with dehydration, can be excluded.

Anemia is now recognized to be more common than previously thought and may affect over 25% of COPD patients. The presence of anemia indicates a poor prognosis in COPD patients receiving long-term oxygen treatment.

Screening for α_1-antitrypsin deficiency should be undertaken in patients less than 45 years of age who develop COPD and/or have a strong family history of the disease. Serum concentrations of α_1-antitrypsin below 15–20% of the normal value are highly suggestive of deficiency. These findings should lead to family screening and appropriate counseling.

Electrocardiography. Routine ECG is not required in the assessment of patients with COPD, and is an insensitive technique in the diagnosis of cor pulmonale.

Pulmonary arterial pressure. Patients with chronic hypoxemia may have mild-to-moderate pulmonary hypertension (mean pulmonary arterial pressure 30–45 mmHg). Measurement of pulmonary arterial pressure is not routinely recommended in clinical practice as it does not add any further information beyond that obtained by assessing arterial blood gases.

Differential diagnosis
It is often difficult to differentiate some patients with chronic asthma from those with COPD, and it is often assumed that asthma and COPD coexist in these patients. Other conditions to be considered in the differential diagnosis of COPD are listed in Table 4.5.

TABLE 4.5

Features of COPD and other conditions to be considered in the differential diagnosis

COPD

- Onset in midlife
- Slowly progressive symptoms
- Exposure to risk factors (e.g. tobacco smoking, occupational dust)
- Breathlessness during exercise
- Largely irreversible airflow limitation

Asthma

- Onset in early life
- Variable symptoms
- Particularly variable at night or the early morning
- Associated features of atopy, allergy, rhinitis and eczema
- Family history of atopy/asthma
- Largely reversible airflow limitation

Tuberculosis

- Chest radiograph shows lung infiltrate
- Onset at all ages
- Microbiological confirmation
- High local prevalence of tuberculosis

Bronchiectasis

- Large volumes of purulent sputum
- Associated bacterial infection
- Clubbing
- Coarse crackles on auscultation
- Bronchial wall thickening and bronchial dilatation seen on chest radiograph or CT scan

Congestive cardiac failure

- Presence of fine basal crackles on auscultation
- Dilated heart and evidence of pulmonary edema on chest radiograph
- Lung function tests indicate restrictive defect (see Figure 4.3, page 47)

Obliterative bronchiolitis

- Onset at a younger age
- Non-smokers affected
- May have history of rheumatoid arthritis or fume exposure
- Mosaic pattern on expiratory CT scan

CT, computed tomography

Key points – lung function tests

- Spirometry is the most important measurement in COPD and is essential for diagnosis. Forced expiratory volume in 1 second (FEV_1) and forced vital capacity (FVC) are recorded in absolute values (liters) and also as a percentage of the predicted values for the individual depending on age, height, sex and ethnic origin.
- An FEV_1 over 80% of the predicted value is considered to be normal.
- Airflow obstruction is defined as an FEV_1 below 80% of the predicted value and an FEV_1:FVC ratio of less than 70%.
- A standardized technique must be employed in spirometry assessment. It is critical that the expiratory flow trace reaches a plateau to prove that the patient has reached the FVC.
- Reversibility testing to bronchodilators is useful in differential diagnosis to distinguish those with marked reversibility indicative of asthma.
- There is no standard assessment of reversibility; generally, however, an improvement in FEV_1 of both 200 mL and 15% over the baseline is interpreted as a positive result.
- Peak expiratory flow rate is not the best assessment of airway obstruction in COPD and may underestimate the degree of airway obstruction.
- Further tests of lung volumes and the diffusing capacity in the lung for carbon monoxide may be helpful in some cases.

Key references

Borg G. Psychophysical basis of perceived exertion. *Med Sci Sports Exerc* 1982;84:377–81.

Gibson GJ, MacNee W. Chronic obstructive pulmonary disease: investigations and assessment of severity. *Eur Respir Mon* 2006;38: 24–40.

Global initiative for chronic Obstructive Lung Disease. Assessment. *Global Strategy for the Diagnosis, Management, and Prevention of Chronic Obstructive Pulmonary Disease. NHLBI/WHO Workshop Report.* Updated 2008. www.goldcopd.com/Guidelineitem. asp?l1=2&l2=1&intId=2003 Accessed 12 January 2009.

Guyatt GH, Berman LB, Townsend M et al. A measure of quality of life for clinical trials in chronic lung disease. *Thorax* 1987;42:773–8.

Jones PW, Quirk FH, Baveystock CM, Littlejohns P. A self-complete measure for chronic airflow limitation: the St. George's questionnaire. *Am Rev Respir Dis* 1992;147:832–8.

McGavin CR, Artvinli M, Naoe H. Dyspnoea, disability and distance walked: a comparison of estimates of exercise performance in respiratory disease. *BMJ* 1978;2:241–3.

Noseda A, Carpeiaux JP, Schmerber J. Dyspnoea assessed by visual analogue scale in patients with obstructive lung disease during progressive and high intensity exercise. *Thorax* 1992;47:363–8.

Rodriquez-Roisin R, MacNee W. Pathophysiology of chronic obstructive pulmonary disease. *Eur Respir Mon* 2006;38:177–200.

Singh SJ, Morgan MDL, Scott SC et al. The development of the shuttle walking test of disability in patients with chronic airway obstruction. *Thorax* 1992;47:1019–24.

No features specific for COPD are seen on a plain posterior-anterior chest radiograph. The features usually described are those of severe emphysema. However, no abnormalities may be present, even in patients with very appreciable disability. Recent improvements in imaging techniques, particularly the advent of computed tomography (CT) and, more recently, high-resolution CT (HRCT), have provided more sensitive means of diagnosing emphysema in life.

Plain chest radiography

The most reliable radiographic signs of emphysema can be classified by their causes of overinflation, vascular changes and bullae.

Overinflation of the lungs results in the following radiographic features:
- a low, flattened diaphragm (Figure 5.1): the diaphragm is abnormally low if the border of the diaphragm in the midclavicular line is at or below the anterior end of the seventh rib; and the diaphragm is flattened if the perpendicular height from a line drawn between the costal and cardiophrenic angles to the border of the diaphragm is less than 1.5 cm
- increased retrosternal airspace, visible on the lateral film at a point 3 cm below the manubrium when the horizontal distance from the posterior surface of the aorta to the sternum exceeds 4.5 cm
- an obtuse costophrenic angle on the posterior-anterior or lateral chest radiograph
- an inferior margin of the retrosternal airspace 3 cm or less from the anterior aspect of the diaphragm.

Vascular changes associated with emphysema result from loss of alveolar walls and are shown on the plain chest radiograph by:
- a reduction in the size and number of pulmonary vessels, particularly at the periphery of the lung

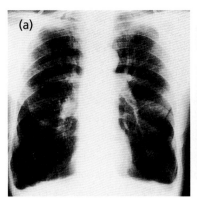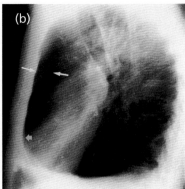

Figure 5.1 Plain chest radiographs of generalized emphysema particularly affecting the lower zones. (a) Posterior-anterior radiograph showing a low, flat diaphragm (below the anterior ends of the seventh ribs), obtuse costophrenic angles and reduced vessel markings in lower zones, which are transradiant. (b) Lateral radiograph showing a low, flat and inverted diaphragm and widened retrosternal transradiancy (white arrows) that approaches the diaphragm inferiorly (blue arrows).

- vessel distortion, producing increased branching angles, excess straightening or bowing of vessels
- areas of transradiancy.

Assessment of the vascular loss in emphysema clearly depends on the quality of the radiograph. A generally increased transradiancy may simply be due to overexposure.

The development of right ventricular hypertrophy produces non-specific cardiac enlargement on the plain chest radiograph. Pulmonary hypertension may be suggested, taking measurements from the plain chest radiograph of the width of the right descending pulmonary artery, just below the right hilum, where the borders of the artery are delineated against the air in the lungs laterally and the right main-stem bronchus medially. The upper limit of the normal range of the width of the artery in this area is 16 mm in men and 15 mm in women. This increase in pulmonary artery size is often associated with a rapid diminution in the size of the vessels as they branch into the pulmonary periphery. Although these measurements can be used to detect the presence or absence of pulmonary hypertension, they cannot accurately predict the level of the pulmonary artery pressure and they are not felt to be particularly sensitive.

Bullae. Focal areas of transradiancy surrounded by hairline walls represent bullae.

Computed tomography

CT scanning has been used to detect and quantify emphysema. Techniques can be divided into those that use visual assessment of low-density areas on the CT scan, which can be either semiquantitative or quantitative, and those that use CT lung density to quantify areas of low X-ray attenuation. These two techniques are usually employed to measure macroscopic or microscopic emphysema, respectively.

A visual assessment of emphysema on CT scanning (Figure 5.2) reveals:

- areas of low attenuation without obvious margins or walls
- attenuation and pruning of the vascular tree
- abnormal vascular configurations.

The sign that correlates best with areas of macroscopic emphysema is an area of low attenuation. Visual inspection of the CT scan can locate areas of macroscopic emphysema, though a visual assessment of the extent of macroscopic emphysema is insensitive and subjective with high intra- and inter-observer variability.

It is possible to distinguish the various types of emphysema using HRCT, particularly when the changes are not severe. The distinction

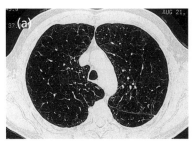 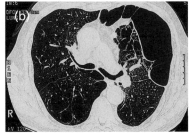

Figure 5.2 High-resolution computed tomography scans of the lungs. (a) Diffuse panlobular emphysema. (b) More patchy centrilobular emphysema with bullae.

depends on the distribution of the lesions: those of centrilobular emphysema are patchy and prominent in the upper zones; whereas those of panlobular emphysema are diffuse throughout the lung zones.

Measurement of lung density on CT in terms of Hounsfield units (a scale of X-ray attenuation where bone is +1000 Hounsfield units, water is 0 Hounsfield units and air is –1000 Hounsfield units) provides a more quantitative way of assessing emphysema (Figure 5.3), particularly at the microscopic level.

A quantitative approach to assessing macroscopic emphysema has been taken by highlighting picture elements, or pixels, within the lung fields in a predetermined low density range, between –910 and –1000 Hounsfield units, which is known as the 'density mask' technique.

If CT scanning is to be used to measure microscopic emphysema, care should be taken to standardize the scanning conditions, particularly the lung volume, and to calibrate the CT scanner, since these factors affect CT lung density. These techniques have not, as yet, been sufficiently standardized for use in clinical practice, but density measurements have been shown to correlate with morphometric measurements of distal airspace size in resected lungs.

Whether a bulla is detected on a chest radiograph depends on its size and the degree to which it is obscured by overlying lung. CT scanning is much more sensitive than plain chest radiography in detecting bullae and can be used to determine their number, size and position.

Echocardiography

Echocardiography has been used to assess the right ventricle and to detect pulmonary hypertension in COPD. However, overinflation of the chest increases the retrosternal airspace, which therefore transmits sound waves poorly, making echocardiography difficult in patients with COPD. Nevertheless, an adequate examination can be achieved in 65–85% of patients with COPD.

Two-dimensional echocardiography has been used in the investigation of right ventricular dimensions and is superior to clinical methods since it shows reasonable correlations between pulmonary artery pressure and various right ventricular dimensions.

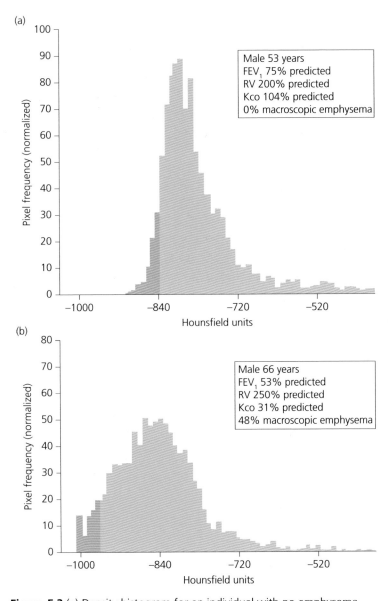

Figure 5.3 (a) Density histogram for an individual with no emphysema.
(b) Density histogram for a patient with severe emphysema. The darker
area represents the lowest 5% of the distribution. FEV$_1$, forced expiratory
volume in 1 second; Kco, carbon monoxide transfer coefficient;
RV, residual volume.

Pulsed-wave Doppler echocardiography has been used to assess the ejection flow dynamics of the right ventricle in patients with pulmonary hypertension. The parameters measured include: acceleration time (in milliseconds), which is defined as the time between the onset of ejection to peak velocity; right ventricular pre-ejection time (in milliseconds), which is the interval from the Q wave of the ECG to the beginning of the forward flow; and right ventricular ejection time (in milliseconds), which is the interval between the onset and termination of flow in the right ventricular outflow tract. Although the pulsed-wave Doppler technique is useful in differentiating patients with an elevated pulmonary arterial pressure from those with normal pulmonary arterial pressure, it is not as accurate as the continuous-wave Doppler technique in assessing pulmonary arterial pressure.

The best technique for non-invasive evaluation of pulmonary arterial pressure is continuous-wave Doppler echocardiography; the tricuspid gradient assessed in this way can be used to calculate the right ventricular systolic pressure. The technique estimates the pressure gradient across the regurgitant jet recorded by Doppler ultrasound. The maximum velocity of the regurgitant jet is measured from the continuous-wave Doppler recordings, and the simplified Bernoulli

---

Key points – imaging

- No features on plain chest radiography are specific for COPD; the features usually described are those of severe emphysema. However, there may be no abnormality even in patients with marked disability.
- Computed tomography (CT) can be used to quantify emphysema, either by visual assessment of high-resolution scanning or by CT lung density measurements.
- CT scanning is the best way to detect and assess bullous disease.
- Echocardiography, particularly continuous-wave Doppler echocardiography, can be used to assess pulmonary arterial pressure in patients with COPD.

equation is used to calculate the maximum pressure gradient between the right ventricle and the right atrium as:

$$P_{RV} - P_{RA} = 4v^2$$

where P_{RV} and P_{RA} are the right ventricular and right atrial pressures and v is the maximum velocity.

The right atrial pressure is estimated from clinical examination of the jugular venous pressure. There is still debate as to whether this technique is sufficiently sensitive and reproducible to monitor longitudinal changes in pulmonary arterial pressure and the effects of therapeutic interventions, particularly in patients with COPD.

Key references

Coxson HO, Rogers RM. New concepts in the radiological concepts of COPD. *Semin Respir Crit Care Med* 2005;26:211–20.

Freidman PJ. Imaging studies in emphysema. *Proc Am Thorac Soc* 2008;5:494–500.

O'Brien C, Guest PJ, Hill SL, Stockley RA. Physiological and radiological characterization of patients diagnosed with chronic obstructive pulmonary disease in primary care. *Thorax* 2000;55:635–42.

Cigarette smoking is the single most important factor in the development of COPD. Smoking cessation is therefore the single most important therapeutic intervention. The earlier a smoker quits, the more advantages accrue.

Most cigarette smokers (> 85%) are addicted to nicotine and experience a well-defined withdrawal syndrome to varying degrees following cessation (Table 6.1). These symptoms peak in the first few days following cessation and gradually decrease after 2–3 weeks. Episodes of craving, which may be intense, may recur for many years; they are often initiated by environmental or behavioral cues associated with smoking. It is important that smokers are informed that these cravings will subside with or without relapse to smoking.

Smoking should not be oversimplified as merely a lifestyle choice, but, owing to the addiction, should be considered as a primary disease

TABLE 6.1

Withdrawal syndrome following smoking cessation*

- Dysphoric or depressed mood
- Insomnia
- Irritability, frustration or anger
- Anxiety
- Difficulty concentrating
- Restlessness
- Decreased heart rate
- Increased appetite or weight gain
- Craving to smoke[†]

*Defined in the *Diagnostic and Statistical Manual of Mental Disorders*. 4th edn. Arlington, Virginia: American Psychiatric Association, 2000.
[†]Not included in the *Diagnostic and Statistical Manual of Mental Disorders* for 'logical reasons', but a characteristic of the syndrome.

entity in itself. In this context, smoking is properly classified as a
chronic, often relapsing, disease. Smoking cessation is thus not simply a
matter of personal choice, but is a legitimate therapeutic intervention,
the goal of which is to induce a 'remission' in smoking.

Recent data indicate that smokers differ in their biological propensity
to become smokers and that genetic factors may affect their ability to
quit. Therapeutic interventions targeted at individual smokers'
susceptibilities are currently under intensive investigation. Available
therapies can nevertheless help a substantial minority of smokers to quit.

Among adult smokers, approximately 70% wish to stop smoking,
and as many as 45% make a serious attempt in each year. Despite this,
only 2% of smokers successfully quit spontaneously in a year. Simple
physician advice to quit can increase these rates to 5–6%. Additional
non-pharmacological support, which can include behavioral, cognitive
and motivational support, as well as pharmacological therapy can
further increase quit rates. Current recommendations are, therefore, that
all physicians establish smoking status as a 'vital sign' at every visit and
undertake appropriate smoking cessation intervention (Figure 6.1).

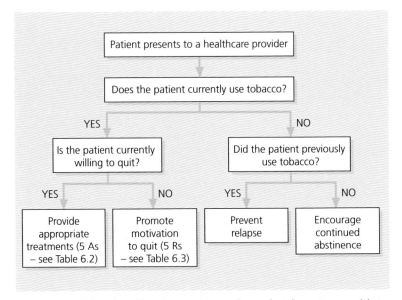

Figure 6.1 Brief antismoking intervention to be undertaken at every visit to
the healthcare provider.

These steps ensure that smokers receive maximum encouragement to quit.

- Brief interventions should be implemented in all practices.
- Intensive interventions are appropriate for many COPD patients. Each practitioner caring for COPD patients should have the option of referring patients for intensive intervention.
- System approaches ensure smoking cessation intervention is integrated into each practice and is fully supported by the healthcare system.

Brief interventions

Brief interventions can be highly effective for many smokers. The five As (Table 6.2) provide key steps for a brief intervention that can be

TABLE 6.2

The five As for physician intervention

Ask

Implement a system that ensures that tobacco use is queried and documented for every patient at every clinic visit

Advise

In a clear, strong and personalized manner, urge all tobacco users to quit

Assess

Ask every tobacco user if he or she is willing to attempt to quit at this time (e.g. within the next 30 days)

Assist

Help the patient make a quit plan, provide practical counseling and intra-treatment social support, help the patient obtain extra-treatment social support, recommend use of approved pharmacotherapy (except in special circumstances) and provide supplementary materials

Arrange

Schedule follow-up contact, either in person or by telephone accomplished within a few minutes and can be tailored to the needs of each smoker.

Smokers not yet ready to quit should be provided with a brief intervention to increase motivation. This should be sympathetic and non-confrontational, and should provide patient-specific information. The five Rs can provide guidance in this respect (Table 6.3). The patient should also understand that the physician is working in their best interest and will be prepared to offer appropriate smoking cessation counseling when the patient is ready.

Every smoker ready to attempt to quit should be offered the highest probability of success. Non-pharmacological support, pharmacological treatment and follow-up all contribute to success.

Behavioral support. Data show clearly that the more behavioral support offered the more likely a smoker is to quit. Many smokers, however, will not attend intensive behavioral programs. Brief behavioral help is therefore appropriate for most individuals and a number of approaches are shown in Table 6.4. Telephone quit-lines also have well-demonstrated efficacy and are widely available.

Pharmacological treatment. All smokers making a serious attempt to quit should be offered pharmacological treatment (in the absence of contraindications). Treatment with first-line medicines for smoking cessation can double or triple quit rates compared with those achieved without pharmacological support. Second-line treatments should be considered for smokers who have failed first-line treatment.

First-line treatments for smoking cessation include nicotine replacement therapy, varenicline and bupropion (also known as amfebutamone).

Nicotine replacement therapy is available in several formulations: polacrilex gum, transdermal systems, inhaler, nasal spray and lozenges. Several other formulations are under investigation. All are similar in efficacy and approximately double quit rates compared with placebo, though they differ in clinical use. This form of therapy has been in use the longest and many over-the-counter formulations are available. Many patients will therefore have had prior experience with these treatments.

TABLE 6.3

The five Rs for smoker motivation

Relevance

- Personalize the reasons to quit. This may include issues in addition to COPD

Risks

- Acute: dyspnea, cough, exacerbations, increased carbon monoxide levels
- Chronic: COPD progression, cancer, cardiovascular disease, osteoporosis, peptic ulcer
- Environmental: disease risk to spouse and other household members, increased risk of smoking and of disease in children

Rewards

- Improves health
- Improves self-image, sense of taste and smell
- Saves money
- Sets a good example for children

Roadblocks

- Withdrawal symptoms
- Fear of failure
- Weight gain
- Lack of support
- Depression
- Enjoyment of tobacco

Repetition

- Most smokers make several quit attempts before achieving long-term abstinence; smoking can be regarded as a chronic relapsing condition, but prolonged remissions are possible

The use of nicotine replacement therapy for smoking cessation is based on the pharmacokinetics of nicotine as a psychoactive drug. The

TABLE 6.4

Behavioral support for smokers trying to quit

Help establish a quit plan

- Set a quit date (ideally within 2 weeks)
- Tell family and friends
- Anticipate challenges
- Remove tobacco products

Counseling

- Be aware that abstinence is essential (most smokers who smoke at all after the quit date will relapse to the previous habit)
- Utilize experience from previous quit attempts
- Anticipate challenges
- Avoid alcohol (the most frequent relapses occur with concurrent alcohol)
- Consider the effect of other smokers in the household (supportive, obstructive, prepared to quit too?)

Encourage other support

- Enlist family, friends and coworkers to assist
- Find support groups

Provide educational materials

- Should be available in every clinician's office. Many are available through a variety of agencies

'hit' associated with nicotine depends on both the amount of nicotine that reaches the brain and the rate of rise in the concentration. The peaks not only provide the psychoactive effect of nicotine, but also contribute to both the psychological and the biological reinforcing mechanisms leading to addiction. Withdrawal symptoms are believed to develop when nicotine levels fall below a certain threshold (Figure 6.2). This generally occurs several hours after the last cigarette, as nicotine has a half-life of the order of hours in most individuals. The concept behind nicotine replacement therapy, therefore, is to provide a steady-

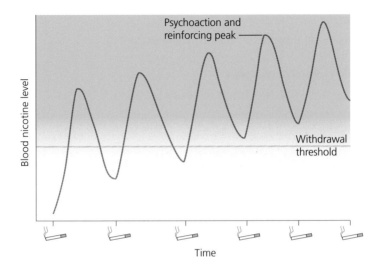

Figure 6.2 Peaks in blood nicotine level provide the psychoactive effect, and contribute to the psychological and biological reinforcing mechanisms leading to addiction. Withdrawal symptoms are believed to develop when the nicotine level falls below a certain threshold.

state level that can protect against the symptoms of withdrawal without providing the reinforcement that contributes to addiction.

Currently available nicotine formulations provide only partial nicotine replacement for most smokers, and none completely prevents withdrawal symptoms, but they do reduce them. More importantly, nicotine replacement therapies increase quit rates. The general strategy for their use is to establish a quit day and to start nicotine replacement on that day. Therapy is then continued for 10 weeks to 6 months. Individual preferences for the various formulations allow the physician some choice in individualizing therapy. The various formulations also have different pharmacokinetics. This is likely to affect their potential to sustain addiction; many individuals have substituted nicotine gum for cigarettes, but remained addicted. It is generally considered, however, that the health hazards associated with the gum are dramatically less than those associated with smoking.

Because the available formulations generally provide incomplete nicotine replacement, there is some possibility for combination therapy.

Several reports suggest that this can offer benefits, though it is an off-label use.

Varenicline is the most recently approved pharmacological agent for smoking cessation. It functions as a partial agonist and is selective for the α4β2 nicotinic receptor. Consistent with its ability to partially activate this receptor, individuals who quit smoking while being treated with varenicline have reduced withdrawal symptoms. In addition, individuals who continue to smoke experience less of the rewarding effects of nicotine, consistent with the antagonism expected of a partial agonist (Figure 6.3). Clinical trials suggest that varenicline can achieve abstinence rates that are three times better than placebo, and that are better than both bupropion and nicotine replacement therapy.

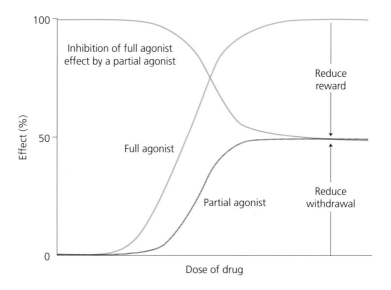

Figure 6.3 The actions of a partial agonist for smoking cessation. A full agonist (green line) results in increasing effect with increasing dose and resembles the effect of nicotine. A partial agonist (red line) results in a partial effect, no matter how much is added. By mimicking the effect of nicotine, varenicline may reduce the effects of withdrawal. In addition, a partial agonist blocks the full effect of a full agonist (blue line) and, in this way, varenicline may reduce the rewarding effects of nicotine.

Varenicline is usually started at a dose of 0.5 mg once daily for 3 days, increased to 0.5 mg twice daily for 3 days and then increased to 1 mg twice daily. The slow increase in dose reduces the incidence of nausea, which is the most common adverse effect. Other relatively common side effects include insomnia and abnormal dreams. Because the drug is primarily excreted unchanged by the kidney, no change in dose is required for concurrent hepatic disease, but a decrease in dose to 0.5 mg/day is recommended in patients with compromised renal function (e.g. creatinine clearance < 30 mL/minute).

Mood and behavioral disturbances have been reported in patients treated with varenicline, including depression, agitation, suicidal thoughts, and aggressive and erratic behavior. It may be difficult to separate some of these symptoms from nicotine withdrawal. The reports have, however, led to a labeling change in the USA, and patients, their families and caregivers should be alerted to monitor for these neuropsychiatric symptoms.

There are no data, as yet, regarding the combination of varenicline with other medications for smoking cessation.

Bupropion also acts directly on the central nervous system, and is in use as an antidepressant. It approximately doubles quit rates compared with placebo, and may be particularly effective in individuals with a history of depression. Bupropion and nicotine replacement therapy can be used in combination. Bupropion is generally started 1 week before the quit day so that adequate blood levels can be achieved. The usual initial dose is 150 mg once a day and is increased to twice a day after 3 days if tolerated. Bupropion should not be used in individuals at risk of seizures or with a history of bulimia or anorexia, and should not be prescribed for patients who are currently receiving bupropion for the treatment of depression.

Second-line therapies include clonidine and nortriptyline. Clonidine has been evaluated in several clinical trials and, though it is not approved and the individual trials did not consistently show statistically significant benefits, a meta-analysis supports its use. Physicians comfortable with this medication can consider it an aid to smoking cessation.

The antidepressant nortriptyline has also been evaluated in several clinical trials, which have shown clinical efficacy. This agent is available as an antidepressant and can therefore be used off-label for smoking cessation by physicians comfortable with its use.

Follow-up evaluations. Success in smoking cessation is closely linked to follow-up. All smokers making a serious attempt to quit should therefore be offered follow-up assessment. Such assessments can deal with specific problems related to cessation and medication use, and can provide behavioral support. Follow-up 1–2 weeks after the quit day is generally recommended. Additional follow-ups can also be beneficial.

Intensive interventions

Intensive interventions are more elaborate than the brief interventions described above. Generally speaking, they require trained counselors and can be conducted either as individual or group sessions. Most often multiple sessions are necessary. Only a minority of smokers referred for intensive programs will attend. Such programs can, however, provide important support for many smokers, and every practitioner should be able to refer patients for intensive intervention.

Key points – smoking cessation

- Smoking should be regarded as a primary chronic relapsing disease.
- All serious attempts to quit should be maximally supported with behavioral and pharmacological interventions.
- Repeated efforts by the physician are required to provide sufficient motivation for a quit attempt.
- Relapses are common, and should engender repeated attempts.
- Smoking cessation activities should be an integrated part of every medical practice.

Approach to system integration

Cigarette smoking should be regarded as a primary disease, and its treatment should be integrated into each healthcare system. This should include adequate training of personnel to interview patients for smoking status as a 'vital sign'. The healthcare system should also provide adequate support for smoking cessation efforts and personnel at all levels should be active participants in smoking cessation interventions. Data show that quit rates increase when more personnel at more levels participate in smoking cessation therapy.

Key references

Daughton D, Susman J, Sitorius M et al. Transdermal nicotine therapy and primary care. Importance of counseling, demographic and patient selection factors on one-year quit rates. The Nebraska Primary Practice Smoking Cessation Trial Group. *Arch Fam Med* 1998;7:425–30.

Fiore MC, chair. Treating tobacco use and dependence: 2008 update. www.ncbi.nlm.nih.gov/books/bv.fcgi? rid=hstat2.chapter.28163 Accessed 14 January 2009.

Fiore MC. US public health service clinical practice guideline: treating tobacco use and dependence. *Respir Care* 2000;45:1200–62.

Fiore MC, Bailey WC, Cohen SJ. *Smoking cessation. Guideline technical report no. 18.* Rockville, MD: US Dept of Health and Human Services, Public Health Service, Agency for Health Care Policy and Research. Publication No. AHCPR 97-No4, October 1997.

Rennard SI, Hepp L. Cigarette smoke induced disease. In: Stockley R, Rennard S, Rabe K, Celli B, eds. *Chronic Obstructive Pulmonary Disease.* Oxford: Blackwell Publishing, 2006.

Schwartz JL. *Review and evaluation of smoking cessation methods: the United States and Canada, 1978–1985.* NIH Publication No. 87-2940, 1987:1125–56.

West R, Shiffman S. *Fast Facts – Smoking Cessation.* 2nd edn. Oxford: Health Press Limited, 2007.

Pharmacological treatment: bronchodilators

Rationale and physiology of benefit. Bronchodilators are the first-line treatment for patients with COPD. It may seem paradoxical that COPD, which by definition has at best limited reversibility, is treated with bronchodilators as first-line therapy. However, even small improvements in airflow can make a significant difference to COPD patients.

Most people have some degree of airway smooth muscle tone, including patients with COPD. Thus, normal individuals will often experience a very modest improvement in airflow when given a bronchodilator. Sedentary normal individuals seldom notice any ease in breathing as a result. Patients with COPD, however, for whom the cost of breathing is substantially greater, especially on exercising, often notice significant improvements in the ease with which they breathe with even modest improvements in airflow.

Even in the absence of measurable improvements in airflow, patients with COPD may still derive benefit from bronchodilators. The likely explanation is that airflow in COPD patients is not only compromised, but is irregularly compromised. As a result, the rate at which different portions of the lung empty during exhalation is variable. With increasing respiratory rate, the areas most severely affected become hyperinflated (see Chapter 2). Subtle improvements in airflow, which result in better matching of the rates with which various portions of the lung empty, probably have an important effect on lung volumes, particularly with increasing respiratory rates, even if total airflow is relatively unaffected. This can lead to a gratifying apparent paradox in which a patient has significant clinical improvement in dyspnea on exertion in the absence of any measurable improvement in forced expiratory volume in 1 second (FEV_1) at rest.

Clinical monitoring. In view of the above, all patients with COPD should be treated initially and aggressively with bronchodilators to control symptoms. Their response should be monitored with objective measures of airflow and on the basis of clinical outcomes, such as symptoms and performance. Adequate assessment of clinical response may require exercise challenge. It is common for patients with COPD to restrict their level of activity progressively as the disease worsens. This reduces dyspnea, but at the cost of an increasingly sedentary existence. Treatment with bronchodilators alone is often insufficient to treat such patients. Usually, improvements in physiological function can benefit the patient only if the bronchodilator treatment is used together with an aggressive rehabilitation program (see pages 103–7). Thus, though bronchodilators form first-line therapy in COPD, for their use to be successful they must be integrated into an appropriate management plan, such as that suggested in the Global initiative for chronic Obstructive Lung Disease guidelines (Table 7.1).

In mild COPD ($FEV_1 \geq 80\%$ predicted), patients are unlikely to experience dyspnea. If dyspnea does develop, short-acting bronchodilators can be given on an as-needed basis. Since dyspnea is most likely to develop following exercise, it may be prudent to give bronchodilators before exertion in order to facilitate a greater level of activity rather than to administer them following exertion. Long-acting bronchodilators may help to maintain high levels of activity on a regular basis.

For patients with moderate COPD, regular treatment with one or more bronchodilators is recommended. Long-acting bronchodilators are appealing, as optimizing airflow for as long as possible throughout the day and night seems advantageous in maximizing performance ability. This treatment should be integrated into an exercise and/or rehabilitation program. Inhaled glucocorticosteroids can be considered. They are most likely to be of benefit as the disease worsens and exacerbation frequency increases.

Classes of bronchodilator. There are three main classes of bronchodilator (Figure 7.1):

- β-agonists
- anticholinergics
- theophylline.

TABLE 7.1

Treatment of stable COPD

GOLD stage	Characteristics	Recommended treatment
All stages		Avoidance of risk factor(s) Influenza vaccination Education of patients about how and when to use treatment Review of treatments prescribed for other conditions
I: mild COPD	FEV_1:FVC < 70% $FEV_1 \geq 80\%$ predicted	As above *plus* Short-acting bronchodilator when needed
II: moderate COPD	FEV_1:FVC < 70% $50\% \leq FEV_1 < 80\%$ predicted	As above *plus* Regular treatment with one or more long-acting bronchodilators plus rehabilitation
III: severe COPD	FEV_1:FVC < 70% $30\% \leq FEV_1 < 50\%$ predicted	As above *plus* Inhaled glucocorticosteroids if repeated exacerbations
IV: very severe COPD	FEV_1:FVC < 70% $FEV_1 < 30\%$ predicted or presence of respiratory failure or right heart failure	As above *plus* Long-term oxygen therapy if chronic respiratory failure present Consider surgical treatments

FEV_1, forced expiratory volume in 1 second, FVC, forced vital capacity; GOLD, Global initiative for chronic Obstructive Lung Disease.
Based on *Global Strategy for the Diagnosis, Management, and Prevention of Chronic Obstructive Pulmonary Disease. NHLBI/WHO Workshop Report.* Updated 2008.

Both short-acting and long-acting agents or formulations are available (or will be available) in all three classes.

β-agonists act as bronchodilators by acting on the $β_2$-subclass of β-agonist receptors in airway smooth muscle thereby increasing cyclic adenosine monophosphate (cAMP) levels and thus decreasing airway

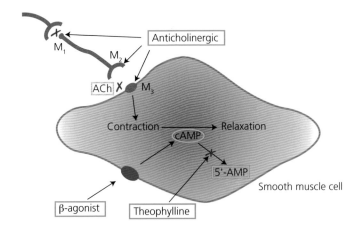

Figure 7.1 Mechanisms of action of bronchodilators: anticholinergics block muscarinic receptors so that acetylcholine is unable to act upon them; β-agonists increase levels of cAMP; theophylline blocks conversion of cAMP to 5'-AMP. M_1, M_2 and M_3 are three distinct types of muscarinic cholinergic receptors. ACh, acetylcholine; AMP, adenosine monophosphate; cAMP, cyclic AMP.

smooth muscle tone. β-agonists can act on β-receptors on other cell types as well (e.g. the heart). By relaxing vascular smooth muscle, they can increase blood flow to relatively poorly ventilated areas and may thus cause a reduction in oxygenation in some settings. Effects on airway epithelial cells and inflammatory cells may be beneficial (see below), but the clinical importance of all these non-bronchodilator effects remains uncertain.

A variety of β-agonists are available in a number of formulations (Table 7.2). They fall roughly into two classes: short-acting and long-acting. Most of the commonly used β-agonists are relatively selective for the β_2-receptor subtype. As a result, they have relatively fewer cardiac side effects than the older, non-selective β-agonists such as isoproterenol, as the most important β-receptors in the heart are β_1-receptors. However, because the heart has some β_2-receptors, no selective agent will be entirely free of cardiac effects.

Short-acting β-agonists. Most short-acting β-agonists have a relatively rapid onset of action, achieving measurable bronchodilation within

5 minutes and a maximal effect in about 30 minutes (Figure 7.2). The effect of these agents generally wanes after 2 hours, and the often-stated 4-hour duration of action is somewhat optimistic. As a result, for regular use, these agents must be administered 4–6 times daily.

The most widely used agent is salbutamol, also known as albuterol (salbutamol is the recommended international non-proprietary name favored by the World Health Organization, but albuterol is the generic name in the USA). It is available in a number of formulations, including metered-dose inhaler formulations and nebulized solutions. Administration via a nebulizer may be appropriate for patients with extremely limited airflows and for individuals who cannot coordinate the use of a metered-dose inhaler. Many patients seem to derive benefit from the ritual aspects of applying the nebulizer mask. In some countries, patients prefer nebulizer therapy because it is covered to a greater degree by their healthcare insurance than metered-dose inhaler formulations.

Salbutamol (albuterol) is a chiral molecule and most preparations are racemic (i.e. mixtures of the levo and dextro forms). Only the levo form interacts with the β_2-receptor to have a beneficial effect and it has been suggested that the dextro form contributes to the adverse effects. Preparations of the levo form alone, which may reduce adverse side effects are available both as a metered-dose inhaler and as a nebulized solution.

β-agonists have a number of systemic side effects due to the total absorbed dose, including ventricular contractions, palpitations, tachycardia, tremor, sleep disturbances and hypokalemia. While topical deposition in the airway by inhalation increases the therapeutic index, drug that is deposited in the mouth and swallowed can result in side effects without local benefit. Such side effects can be reduced by the use of spacers or other devices that decrease oral deposition of the drug.

Salbutamol (albuterol) is also available for oral use. As might be expected, oral administration results in a considerably higher systemic dose than the same dose delivered to the lungs by inhalation. As a result, the side effects of tachycardia and tremor are more common, so oral dosing is reserved for highly selected patients. Slow-release oral

91

TABLE 7.2

Common β-agonist bronchodilator formulations

Drug	Inhaler	Nebulizer solution
Fenoterol	100–200 µg MDI	1 mg/mL
Salbutamol (albuterol)	100 µg, 200 µg MDI and DPI	5 mg/mL
Levalbuterol	45 µg MDI	0.63, 1.25 mg in 3 mL
Terbutaline	400 µg, 500 µg MDI	–
Formoterol	4.5–12 µg MDI and DPI	20 µg in 2 mL
Arformoterol	–	15 µg in 2 mL
Salmeterol	25–50 µg MDI and DPI	–

DPI, dry-powder inhaler; MDI, metered-dose inhaler.

formulations of salbutamol (albuterol) permit its use as a long-acting preparation, but do not alter the pharmacokinetics of the drug itself.

Long-acting β-agonists. Two long-acting β-agonist bronchodilators are available: salmeterol and formoterol (eformoterol). Both are long-acting for pharmacokinetic reasons. Salmeterol interacts with two sites on the β-adrenergic receptor: the active site, to activate adenyl cyclase and thus cause cAMP production; and a second site that allows the drug to remain bound to the receptor and thus to have a long duration of action. The long duration of action of formoterol is probably due to its high lipophilicity; it binds to the cell membrane and remains there as a reservoir. Both drugs have a duration of action of 12 hours (see Figure 7.2), making them appropriate for twice-daily dosing. A preparation containing only the (R,R) enantiomer of formoterol, arformoterol, is available for administration via a nebulizer. The onset of action of formoterol is similar to that of salbutamol (albuterol). Salmeterol, however, has a much slower onset of action, achieving bronchodilation within 15–30 minutes and a maximal effect within 2 hours.

Anticholinergic agents affect cholinergic transmission, which is critical in maintaining normal airway smooth muscle tone.

Oral	Injectable	Duration of action (hours)
0.05% (syrup)	–	4–6
5 mg pill; 0.024% syrup	0.1 and 0.5 mg/vial	4–6
–	–	5–8
2.5, 5 mg	0.2 and 0.25 mg/vial	4–6
–	–	≥ 12
–	–	≥ 12
–	–	≥ 12

M_1 muscarinic receptors mediate neural transmission in the vagal ganglia, and M_3 muscarinic receptors at the neuromuscular junctions mediate smooth muscle contraction. Blockade of these receptors, particularly the M_3 receptors, can antagonize normal airway tone and thus result in bronchodilation. M_2 receptors have a feedback control function and may attenuate vagal activity.

Atropine has a modest bronchodilator effect, but is seldom used because of its other systemic effects. The anticholinergic agents most commonly used to achieve bronchodilation are quaternary amines (Table 7.3). When inhaled, these agents are absorbed very poorly, resulting in a high degree of local activity and a very low systemic side-effect profile. Ipratropium bromide is most widely used. It has an onset of action slightly slower than salbutamol, with a bronchodilator effect in 10 minutes, a near-maximal effect in 30 minutes and a duration of action of 4–6 hours (see Figure 7.2). It is available in a metered-dose inhaler and as a nebulized solution. The approved dose in most countries (42 µg or 2 puffs every 6 hours) is probably not at the top of the dose–response curve. As a result, improved bronchodilation and clinical effect can often be achieved with increased doses, and routine administration of 3 or 4 puffs has been suggested and is widely used.

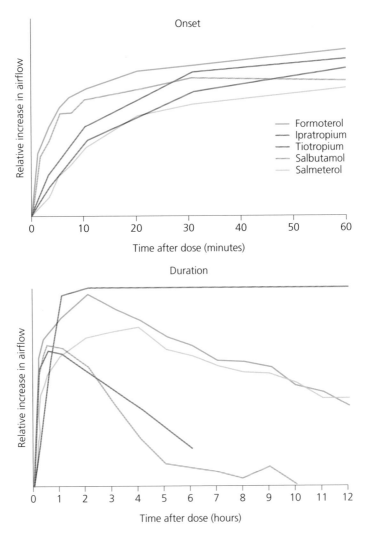

Figure 7.2 Onset and duration of action of bronchodilators.

Interestingly, while the bronchodilator effect of ipratropium bromide is clearly shorter than that of salmeterol, both drugs result in a similar degree of improvement in exercise performance 6 hours after administration. This would be consistent with ipratropium bromide improving lung volumes and reducing dynamic hyperinflation over and above its ability to improve airflow.

TABLE 7.3
Amine anticholinergic bronchodilators

Drug	Metered-dose /dry-powder inhaler (µg)	Nebulizer (mg)	Oral (mg)	Duration of action (hours)
Atropine sulfate*	–	2.0	–	–
Ipratropium bromide	40–80	0.25–0.5	–	6–8
Tiotropium	18	–	–	24–36

*The intravenous atropine preparation has been administered by nebulizer; it is not currently used, as it has adverse systemic effects.

Tiotropium is a long-acting anticholinergic bronchodilator. It dissociates relatively rapidly from the M_2 muscarinic receptor, giving it some selectivity for the M_1 and M_3 receptors. Whether this is of clinical significance is unclear. Its long duration of action is due to its prolonged association with the M_1 and M_3 receptors. Its onset of action is slower than that of ipratropium bromide, but its duration of action is noticeably longer (see Figure 7.2). A bronchodilator effect is still detectable after 36 hours, and the maximal bronchodilator effect accumulates over the first few days of administration. Its duration of action makes it appropriate for once-daily use.

The side effects of anticholinergic agents in clinical use are generally mild and include dry mouth and a metallic taste. Closed-angle glaucoma may develop if drug is deposited in the eye. Men with prostate disease should be monitored for urinary tract effects, but these are uncommon. In patients with asthma, paradoxical bronchoconstriction can occur. A post hoc meta-analysis raised questions about potential increased cardiovascular mortality in patients treated with anticholinergic agents. However, a subsequent 4-year prospective trial of nearly 6000 patients comparing tiotropium with placebo found a decrease in cardiovascular events and a decrease in overall mortality that approached statistical significance in the tiotropium-treated group.

Theophylline is ineffective when administered topically as a bronchodilator and is usually used orally, though it can be administered rectally. Intravenous formulations are no longer routinely used. Theophylline has several mechanisms of action, including inhibition of adenosine receptors and inhibition of multiple species of phosphodiesterase. The mechanism that leads to bronchodilatation is unclear. The traditional concept of phosphodiesterase inhibition leading to increases in cAMP and bronchodilatation has been called into question.

A number of theophylline preparations are available. Theophylline USP (*United States Pharmacopeia*) is comparatively inexpensive, but has a relatively short duration of action. It is cleaved by hepatic enzymes, which can be induced by a variety of stimuli; this leads to marked variations in theophylline clearance between patients and even in a given patient with changes in clinical state. Slow-release theophylline preparations for use once or twice daily provide steadier blood levels and are easier to use clinically. However, theophylline has major adverse side effects, which limit its use. These include: central nervous system effects leading to nausea, vomiting and seizures; arrhythmias; relaxation of the lower gastroesophageal sphincter, causing or worsening gastroesophageal reflux; diarrhea; and headaches. Drug–drug interactions are common and further complicate use in clinical practice.

Many clinicians routinely check theophylline blood levels as toxic effects can be observed at levels only slightly above the traditional therapeutic range of 10–20 µg/mL. Recent practice, however, has been to use theophylline at relatively low doses, maintaining blood levels in the 5–10 µg/mL range. This range is often associated with a satisfying clinical response and has an increased safety margin. A further reason for repeated testing is that, as noted above, theophylline is metabolized by the liver, and hepatic clearance can change, resulting in varying blood levels despite constant dosing and good compliance.

Theophylline can also be combined with β-agonist bronchodilators (with which cAMP levels may be raised synergistically) and with ipratropium bromide.

Combination therapy. It is possible to combine bronchodilators from different classes. While some studies have suggested that a maximal bronchodilator effect can be achieved with a single agent given at sufficiently high dose, several large clinical trials have demonstrated an improvement in bronchodilator effect when a combination of β-agonist and anticholinergic bronchodilators are administered. A commercially available combination of salbutamol and ipratropium bromide (Combivent) has achieved widespread clinical acceptance. Ipratropium bromide and tiotropium can also be used in combination with long-acting β-agonist bronchodilators.

Non-bronchodilator effects of bronchodilators. It is likely that all drugs used to achieve bronchodilatation have a number of other effects. The clinical importance of these non-bronchodilator effects remains undefined.

Long-acting β-agonist bronchodilators and both long- and short-acting anticholinergic bronchodilators have been associated with a reduction in the frequency of COPD exacerbations. The mechanisms by which such an effect might be mediated are unclear. However, salmeterol has direct effects on airway epithelial cells that may mitigate epithelial damage secondary to bacterial infection. β-agonists may inhibit the activity of inflammatory cells and act on blood vessels to reduce the formation of and accelerate the clearance of edema. Anticholinergic agents also have the potential for anti-inflammatory action by inhibiting the release of inflammatory mediators.

Theophylline may also have anti-inflammatory actions in addition to its bronchodilator activity. It can improve diaphragmatic muscle contractility and may have other benefits, including a positive inotropic effect and a mild diuretic effect. In some studies, patients have reported subjective benefits from theophylline out of proportion to its modest bronchodilator activity.

The potential effects of bronchodilators on disease progression are discussed on page 101.

Other pharmacological treatment options

Glucocorticosteroids. Oral corticosteroids should be avoided if at all possible in the management of stable COPD (Table 7.4). Corticosteroid-induced side effects are relatively common and can

TABLE 7.4

Use of glucocorticosteroids in COPD

Systemic

- May be used for short-term treatment (7–14 days) during exacerbations
- Avoid chronic use
- No rationale for a therapeutic challenge

Inhaled

- Modest bronchodilator effect
- Reduce exacerbation frequency/severity
- Improve health status
- No effect on rate of decline in FEV_1

FEV_1, forced expiratory volume in 1 second.

be devastating in COPD patients. Corticosteroid myopathy may further compromise individuals already relatively unable to exercise. Corticosteroid-induced osteoporosis may lead to fractures, which not only compromise mobility but also, if they occur in the spine or ribs, may lead to chest-wall splinting and an increased risk of pneumonia. Chronic administration of oral corticosteroids has been associated with increased mortality in COPD patients. However, systemic corticosteroids may be of benefit during COPD exacerbations (see below). Treatment should be stopped after 7–14 days.

Inhaled corticosteroids may improve airflow. The mechanisms underlying this effect are unclear, but a reduction in airway edema has been suggested. It may take several weeks or even as long as 6 months for the benefits of this treatment to be observed. Generally speaking, the improvement in airflow, if there is any, is much less than that achieved with bronchodilators, averaging about 50 mL compared with 200–300 mL achievable with bronchodilators (see above).

Inhaled corticosteroids also reduce the frequency and severity of exacerbations. This decrease appears to be associated with a beneficial effect on health status (quality of life), which is reasonable, as COPD exacerbations are associated with a worsening in health status. Several large studies have demonstrated a statistically significant benefit in terms of both exacerbations and health status. The effect on exacerbations is generally due to the effect in the most severely affected patients who experience the most frequent exacerbations, although milder cases may also benefit. Inhaled glucocorticosteroids should therefore be considered for patients experiencing frequent exacerbations, particularly if they are already receiving maximal bronchodilator therapy.

The adverse effects of inhaled corticosteroids are far fewer than those associated with systemic administration. Systemic effects, including effects on bone density and skin fragility, are observed with some preparations. Agents that are cleared more rapidly from the circulation have fewer systemic side effects. Local side effects include thrush and dysphonia. Recent clinical trials have shown an increased incidence of pneumonia in patients randomized to inhaled corticosteroids. However, these events have not been well characterized and their clinical importance is unclear.

Two combinations of a long-acting β-agonist and inhaled corticosteroid are currently available: salmeterol plus fluticasone (Seretide) and formoterol plus budesonide (Symbicort). In contrast to COPD, where they may be used independently, long-acting β-agonists are approved for use in asthma only in these combinations. It is likely that collaborative and/or synergistic interactions between β-agonists and corticosteroids can improve asthma control. Whether such benefits also accrue in COPD remains to be determined.

Vaccines. Influenza vaccination is recommended for all elderly patients since it can reduce mortality from influenza by around 50%. It is particularly recommended for patients with COPD. The vaccine is adjusted each year to be effective against the appropriate strains of the virus, and the vaccination is given once in the autumn or twice a year in the autumn and winter. Recent strategies have also advocated immunization of individuals likely to transmit influenza to COPD patients.

Streptococcus pneumoniae is the most common cause of community-acquired pneumonia, and pneumococcal infection is more common in adults over the age of 50. Pneumococcal vaccination has been shown to be beneficial in reducing mortality from streptococcal pneumonia in an elderly population and, by extrapolation, might be expected to be effective in COPD patients. While data regarding the specific use of pneumococcal vaccination in COPD patients are limited, vaccination is recommended.

α_1-antitrypsin augmentation therapy. Patients with severe hereditary α_1-antitrypsin deficiency and established emphysema may be candidates for α_1-antitrypsin replacement therapy. Therapy is expensive and is unavailable in many countries. Data from observational registries suggest that replacement therapy has benefits, but it is not recommended in patients with COPD that is unrelated to α_1-antitrypsin deficiency.

Antibiotic therapy. The continuous, prophylactic use of antibiotics has not been shown to have any significant effect on frequent exacerbations of COPD. Thus, current evidence supports the use of antibiotics to treat the effects of exacerbations of COPD, but their long-term use is not recommended.

Mucolytic agents (ambroxol, carbocisteine, iodinated glycerol) have produced variable results in patients with COPD. Most studies have shown little or no change in lung function or symptoms. A systematic Cochrane collaborative review showed that mucolytic agents reduce episodes of acute-on-chronic bronchitis compared with placebo. Their use, however, still remains controversial.

The mucolytic and antioxidant drug N-acetylcysteine has been shown to reduce the frequency of exacerbations of COPD in patients not taking inhaled corticosteroids.

Antitussives. Cough is a troublesome symptom in COPD, but it does have a protective role and therefore the use of antitussives is contraindicated in stable COPD.

Vasodilators. The rationale for the use of vasodilators is based on the relationship between pulmonary arterial pressure and mortality in

COPD. Numerous vasodilators have been assessed. Most produce small changes in pulmonary arterial pressure, but at the expense of worsening ventilation–perfusion mismatching and therefore worsening gas exchange. There is therefore no indication for vasodilators in COPD.

Other drugs, such as leukotriene antagonists and nedocromil, have not been adequately assessed in COPD and cannot be recommended.

Modification of disease progression

The Lung Health Study was designed to determine whether inhaled ipratropium bromide would alter the rate of decline in lung function in patients with mild COPD. No effect was found, but the dose used (2 puffs three times daily) and relatively poor adherence could have compromised the results.

More recently, the TORCH (TOwards a Revolution in COPD Health) trial evaluated fluticasone, salmeterol, a combination of both drugs and placebo in a 3-year trial involving more than 6000 patients. The primary endpoint, mortality, did not achieve statistical significance, though a strong trend ($p = 0.052$) was observed for the combination therapy compared with placebo (Figure 7.3a). Significant treatment benefits were a reduction in exacerbations, improvement in health status and a reduction in the rate of decline in lung function of 13–16 mL/year.

The UPLIFT (Understanding the Potential Long-term Impacts on Function with Tiotropium) trial also included nearly 6000 patients randomized to receive either tiotropium or placebo in addition to their usual care. Nearly 75% of patients were treated concurrently with an inhaled corticosteroid, a long-acting β-agonist or both. Tiotropium had no effect on the rate of decline in lung function for the groups as a whole. However, it was of significant benefit among those not treated with an inhaled corticosteroid or a long-acting β-agonist. Importantly, tiotropium also had a significant effect in reducing exacerbations and a reduction in mortality was observed at the end of the treatment period (Figure 7.3b), although this benefit lost statistical significance 30 days later, perhaps due to incomplete follow-up.

These two large clinical trials support the aggressive treatment of COPD patients. Reductions in exacerbations and improved health status

101

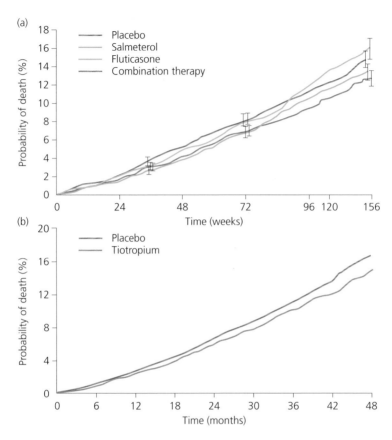

Figure 7.3 Effect of treatment on mortality in COPD. (a) The TORCH trial compared fluticasone, salmeterol, a combination of both drugs and placebo. A trend towards improved survival that did not reach statistical significance ($p = 0.052$) was seen in the group receiving combination treatment compared with placebo. Reproduced from Celli BR et al. 2008, with permission of the American Thoracic Society © 2008. (b) The UPLIFT trial compared tiotropium with placebo in a group of COPD patients, most of whom were treated with an inhaled glucocorticosteroid, a long-acting β-agonist or both. There was a statistically significant reduction in mortality in the tiotropium group at the end of treatment. Follow-up 30 days after discontinuation showed a trend toward improved survival that did not achieve significance ($p = 0.09$). Reproduced from Tashkin DP et al. 2008, with permission from the Massachusetts Medical Society © 2008. All rights reserved.

have clearly been demonstrated. A significant reduction in rate of decline in lung function is encouraging, though the clinical importance of this modest effect remains to be determined. Trends towards improved survival are also encouraging. Furthermore, while the results were not statistically significant, the strong trends observed allay safety concerns that have been raised with respect to bronchodilators and inhaled corticosteroids.

Non-pharmacological treatment

Rehabilitation. Previously, the main management goals in COPD were to prevent a deterioration of the condition, principally by encouraging smoking cessation, and to improve lung function and thus symptoms with bronchodilators. Substantial evidence now suggests that improving health status and functional ability is another attainable goal. The fact that the airflow limitation in COPD is largely irreversible means that the results of pharmacological therapy on lung function are, at best, modest. It is now known that, without changing airflow limitation, pulmonary rehabilitation can still improve both performance and health status.

The principal goals of pulmonary rehabilitation are to reduce symptoms, improve health status, and increase physical and emotional participation in everyday activities. These goals are particularly relevant in the moderate-to-severe stages of COPD, when breathlessness may result in the avoidance of activity. This results in deconditioning of the skeletal muscles, which in turn leads to increasing disability, social isolation and depression. This compounds the problems of dyspnea and lack of fitness, and a vicious circle ensues, resulting in increasing dependence and disability and worsening quality of life (Figure 7.4). The aim of pulmonary rehabilitation is to break this vicious circle of increasing inactivity, breathlessness and physical deconditioning, and improve exercise capacity and functional status.

The main components of a pulmonary rehabilitation program are:
• exercise training
• nutritional counseling
• education.

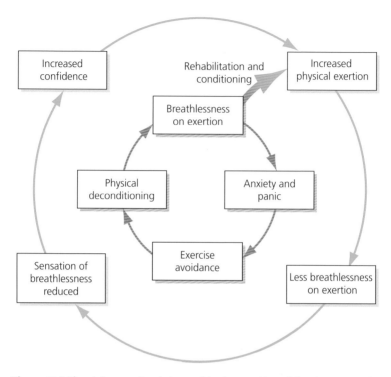

Figure 7.4 The vicious cycle of deconditioning and inactivity that occurs in COPD, and the effect of pulmonary rehabilitation.

At all stages of COPD, patients appear to benefit from exercise training programs, which improve exercise tolerance, symptoms of breathlessness and fatigue. Pulmonary rehabilitation has been assessed in numerous large clinical trials and the benefits are summarized in Table 7.5. Studies suggest that these benefits can be sustained after a single rehabilitation program if the patient maintains the exercise training at home.

The social isolation that accompanies severe COPD can lead to mood disturbances, which may require treatment. It is important to encourage social contact, and contact in the rehabilitation group may provide support. Generally, rehabilitation programs consist of two or three sessions per week for 6–10 weeks and provide a program of exercises that the patient also performs between sessions. The improvement seen with pulmonary rehabilitation programs seems to be long-lasting,

TABLE 7.5

Benefits of pulmonary rehabilitation in COPD

- Improves exercise capacity
- Reduces the perceived intensity of breathlessness
- Improves health-related quality of life
- Reduces the number of hospitalizations and length of hospital stay
- Strength and endurance training of the upper limbs improves arm function
- Benefits extend beyond the immediate period of training
- Improves survival
- Respiratory muscle training is beneficial, especially when combined with general exercise training
- Psychosocial intervention is helpful

persisting for at least a year. Follow-up is beneficial, and occasional repeat sessions have been offered in some centers that provide continuing support.

Rehabilitation involves a multidisciplinary group of healthcare professionals, and has been reported to have benefits in inpatient, outpatient and home settings. Selection criteria for pulmonary rehabilitation are still under investigation. However, benefits are seen in patients with a wide range of disability, though those who are very severely disabled (e.g. those who are chair bound or have an Medical Research Council [MRC] dyspnea grade of 5 [see Table 3.2, page 35]) may not derive any benefit.

It is important that motivated patients are selected for pulmonary rehabilitation. While many believe that inclusion of patients in a pulmonary rehabilitation program should be conditional on their participation in a smoking cessation program, there is no evidence that smokers will benefit less than non-smokers.

Exercise training to recondition skeletal muscles and improve exercise endurance is a key component of pulmonary rehabilitation. Bicycle ergometry and treadmill exercise are both suitable aerobic activities. A number of physiological variables, such as maximum oxygen consumption, maximum heart rate and maximum work performed are measured. A less complex approach utilizes a self-paced walking test (e.g. a 6-minute walking distance). Shuttle walking tests (see page 61) reflect an individual's peak oxygen consumption fairly accurately, provide more information than a 6-minute walking distance and are simpler to perform than a treadmill test.

Exercise training is performed regularly in a form that the patient will be able to continue at home during and after the rehabilitation program. The frequency of exercise varies from daily to weekly, the duration from 10 to 45 minutes and the intensity from 50% of peak oxygen consumption to maximum tolerated. The optimum length of a rehabilitation program has not been determined, and suggestions from randomized controlled trials range from 6 to 10 weeks; however, the longer the program, the more beneficial are the results.

Some programs include training of specific muscle groups, such as the upper limb girdle muscles, and aim to improve the patient's performance of specific tasks associated with daily living. There are no randomized controlled trial data to support the routine use of these exercises, but they may be useful in patients with comorbidity that restricts other forms of exercise and in those with severe COPD who find aerobic exercise too demanding.

The role of respiratory muscle training in pulmonary rehabilitation is still controversial. Training respiratory muscles for both strength and endurance has produced equivocal results in patients with COPD. However, inspiratory muscle training appears to have some additional benefit when undertaken as part of a comprehensive pulmonary rehabilitation program.

Nutritional counseling is based on the fact that the nutritional status of patients with COPD has an important effect on symptoms, disability and prognosis. Being overweight or underweight can be problematic. Around 25% of patients with moderate-to-severe COPD have a reduction in both their body mass index (BMI) and fat-free mass index. A low BMI has been shown to be an independent risk factor for mortality in COPD patients (see Figure 2.4, page 27).

The cause of malnutrition in COPD is complex and may relate to raised levels of various cytokines, including tumor necrosis factor.

Breathlessness while eating can lead to reduced calorie intake and patients should be encouraged to take small, frequent meals. Any problems with dentition should be corrected, and any comorbidity that might result in weight loss should be dealt with. Nutritional support in the form of increased calorie intake is best accompanied by exercise regimens that have an anabolic action. Underweight COPD patients whose nutritional state improves in response to therapy may also improve respiratory muscle strength and survival.

Obese patients with COPD are more likely to have greater impairment of activity and a greater degree of breathlessness than patients of normal weight. These patients should be encouraged to lose weight while taking regular exercise.

Education is included in most pulmonary rehabilitation programs, though its effect is unclear. Smoking cessation is a critical part of pulmonary rehabilitation and may be facilitated by advice and support from the physician (see Chapter 6). Advice should also be given on drug treatment and how to manage exacerbations.

Oxygen therapy. Long-term administration of oxygen therapy ($\geq$ 15 hours/day) has been shown to:
- improve survival
- prevent progression of pulmonary hypertension
- decrease polycythemia.

The UK MRC trial of oxygen, 15 hours/day, showed an increase in 5-year survival from 25% to 41% (compared with no oxygen), and a further trial, the Nocturnal Oxygen Therapy Trial (NOTT), showed that continuous oxygen therapy for a mean period of 17.7 hours/day was more beneficial in terms of survival than use for only 12 hours/day, which conferred no benefit. It is debatable whether oxygen therapy improves health status, but both mood and indices of depression improve.

Oxygen therapy reduces the oxygen costs of breathing and minute ventilation, thus reducing the sensation of breathlessness. It has been given to control severe breathlessness on exercise. Recent data suggest that ambulatory oxygen therapy improves the benefits obtained from exercise training programs.

When given during exercise, oxygen therapy increases walking distance by optimizing oxygen uptake and utilization by the muscles. However, there are no data to indicate whether long-term continuous oxygen therapy improves exercise capacity. Oxygen is administered during exercise to patients who usually fit the criteria for long-term oxygen therapy and to those who experience significant oxygen desaturation during exercise.

The goal of oxygen therapy is to increase the partial pressure of oxygen in arterial blood (PaO_2) to at least 8 kPa (60 mmHg) or to produce a percentage oxygen saturation of arterial blood (SaO_2) of at least 90% to ensure adequate oxygen delivery to vital organs. The treatment should be given to patients with severe COPD and a PaO_2 below 7.3 kPa (55 mmHg) and an SaO_2 below 88%, with or without hypercapnia, as well as to those with a PaO_2 between 7.3 and 8 kPa (55 and 60 mmHg) or an SaO_2 of 89% with evidence of pulmonary hypertension or peripheral edema and polycythemia (hematocrit > 55%). The need for oxygen therapy should be assessed when the patient is in a clinically stable state, at least 6 weeks after the last exacerbation and when other drug therapy has been optimized.

Long-term oxygen therapy is usually provided by an oxygen concentrator via nasal prongs at a flow rate of 2–3 liters/minute. Patients who desaturate during exercise are often told to increase the flow rate during exercise. Portable oxygen can also be provided by liquid oxygen and a portable device or by lightweight oxygen cylinders.

A number of studies have shown that oxygen delivered during exercise (ambulatory oxygen) can reduce the sensation of exercise-induced dyspnea and improve exercise tolerance. However, there is little evidence that the improvement seen in these laboratory studies is translated into improvements in exercise during daily living. In addition, compliance with ambulatory oxygen is poor. There is no good evidence that the use of short bursts of oxygen to relieve breathlessness before or after exercise is beneficial.

Oxygenation during air travel may be insufficient for patients with severe COPD who should, in any case, seek advice about any form of travel. Modern aircraft cabin pressures have oxygen levels equivalent to those 1500–2500 m (5000–8000 feet) above sea level; that is an ambient oxygen pressure of 15–18 kPa (112–135 mmHg). This means that, in a healthy individual, the PaO_2 will decrease from 12 to 8.7 kPa (90 to 65 mmHg) and the SaO_2 from 96% to 90%. This reduction in oxygenation may be hazardous in a patient with severe lung disease and hypoxia unless supplementary oxygen is given during the flight. Patients with COPD are considered able to fly safely, with supplementary oxygen, if:

- their FEV_1 is over 25% of the predicted value
- their PaO_2 during the flight will be over 6.7 kPa (50 mmHg).

Patients with a resting PaO_2 at sea level of over 9.3 kPa (70 mmHg) may safely fly without supplementary oxygen.

If there is any doubt about the advisability of air travel, patients can be referred to a respiratory physician, who may perform a hypoxic challenge in which the patient breathes air with reduced levels of oxygen to assess their likely response to the levels of oxygen present during air travel.

Ventilatory support. The success of non-invasive intermittent positive-pressure ventilation (NIPPV) in patients with respiratory failure during exacerbations of COPD has led to its use in patients with chronic respiratory failure due to severe COPD. Several studies have examined the use of ventilatory support in such patients but have found no convincing evidence that this treatment produces a long-term survival advantage over oxygen therapy alone. Given the conflicting evidence for the use of long-term NIPPV, it cannot be recommended for the routine treatment of patients with chronic respiratory failure due to COPD. However, a combination of NIPPV with long-term oxygen therapy may help some patients with severe daytime hypercapnia.

Surgical treatment

Bullectomy. Some patients with COPD develop large cyst-like spaces, or bullae, in the lungs, which tend to compress the more normal areas of the lung (see Chapter 1, page 16). Removal of bullae that do not contribute to gas exchange may allow decompression of the adjacent lung parenchyma. Bullae can be detected on plain chest radiographs, but are better viewed on CT scans, which also permit the assessment of emphysema in the remaining lung (see Figure 5.2b, page 71). This may be an important determinant of the success of bullectomy.

A range of surgical procedures has been used, including bronchoscopic techniques using laser ablation. In carefully selected patients, such a procedure can improve lung function and symptoms of breathlessness. Patients who would benefit are those who have normal or minimally reduced diffusing capacity in the lung for carbon monoxide (DLco), and those who are not hypoxemic and who have good perfusion in the remaining lung, as assessed by lung perfusion scanning. Individuals less likely to benefit are those with pulmonary hypertension, hypercapnia and severe emphysema in the remaining non-bullous lung.

Lung volume reduction surgery removes emphysematous parts of the lung to decrease overinflation, thus improving the mechanical efficiency of the respiratory muscles, particularly the diaphragm. Lung volume reduction surgery also increases the elastic recoil pressure of the lung, so improving expiratory flow rates. This operation can be performed unilaterally or bilaterally using mediastinotomy or video-assisted thoracoscopy and the mortality rate in good centers is less than 5%.

Selection criteria for those who would derive most benefit are not fully established, although most studies select patients with an FEV_1 less than 35% of the predicted value, a PaO_2 less than 6 kPa (45 mmHg), predominant upper-lobe emphysema on the CT scan and a residual volume of more than 200% of the predicted value. Studies have shown that very severely affected patients with homogeneous disease and an FEV_1 or DLco less than 25% of the predicted value do not benefit; indeed, there is an increased mortality in this group. Conversely, the US National Emphysema Treatment Trial identified individuals with upper-lobe disease and exercise limitation despite optimal medical treatment and rehabilitation as a group of good responders.

Lung volume reduction surgery has been shown to improve FEV_1, decrease total lung capacity, and improve exercise tolerance and quality of life; these effects may last for more than 2 years. In addition, longer-term follow-up has shown that lung volume reduction surgery leads to a greater improvement in maximal work capacity and health-related quality of life, a reduction in exacerbation frequency and improved survival. These beneficial effects are largely seen in those patients with predominant upper-zone emphysema and poor exercise tolerance. Lung volume reduction surgery is expensive and should be reserved for carefully selected patients.

Lung transplantation. In patients with very advanced COPD, lung transplantation has been shown to improve health status and functional capacity, though it does not convey a survival benefit. The main criteria for lung transplantation are FEV_1 less than 35% of the predicted value,

---

Key points – therapy in stable disease

- Bronchodilators are the first-line treatment in COPD; they can be effectively used concurrently and also have beneficial non-bronchodilator effects.
- Inhaled glucocorticosteroids can improve airflow modestly and can reduce the frequency and severity of exacerbations.
- Short courses (7–14 days) of systemic corticosteroids may help following exacerbations, but should not be used over the long term.
- Optimum clinical benefits require an integrated program combining rehabilitation with pharmacotherapy.
- Influenza vaccination is recommended for patients with COPD; there is also some evidence to support pneumococcal vaccination in COPD patients.
- Surgical removal of large bullae and lung volume reduction surgery may improve lung function and symptoms in carefully selected patients.
- Lung transplantation in patients with very advanced COPD improves health status and functional capacity, though it does not convey a survival benefit.
- Rehabilitation has been shown to be beneficial in terms of improving exercise tolerance, symptoms of breathlessness and fatigue in patients with COPD.

PaO_2 less than 7.3–8.0 kPa (55–60 mmHg), $PaCO_2$ over 6.7 kPa (50 mmHg) and secondary pulmonary hypertension. The number of lung transplants is limited by a shortage of donors. Complications after transplantation in patients with COPD include rejection, bronchiolitis obliterans and opportunistic infection. Bronchiolitis occurs in 30% of patients surviving for 5 years and may be fatal. Patients require long-term immunosuppressive therapy.

Key references

Calverley PM, Anderson JA, Celli B et al. Salmeterol and fluticasone propionate and survival in chronic obstructive pulmonary disease. N Engl J Med 2007;356:775–89.

Celli BR, MacNee W. Standards for the diagnosis and treatment of patients with COPD: a summary of the ATS/ERS position paper. Eur Respir J 2004;23:932–46.

Celli BR, Thomas NE, Andersen JA et al. Effect of pharmacotherapy on rate of decline of lung function in COPD: Results from the TORCH Study. Am J Respir Crit Care Med 2008;178:332–8.

Furumoto A, Ohkusa Y, Chen M et al. Additive effect of pneumococcal vaccine and influenza vaccine on acute exacerbation in patients with chronic lung disease. Vaccine 2008;26:4284–9.

Global initiative for chronic Obstructive Lung Disease. Global Strategy for the Diagnosis, Management, and Prevention of Chronic Obstructive Pulmonary Disease. NHLBI/WHO Workshop Report. Updated 2008. www.goldcopd.com/Guidelineitem.asp?l1=2&l2=1&intId=2003 Accessed 12 January 2009.

Mitrouska R, Tzanakis N, Siafakas NM. Oxygen therapy in COPD. Eur Resp Mon 2006;38: 302–12.

National Emphysema Treatment Trial Research Group. A randomized trial comparing lung-volume-reduction surgery with medical therapy for severe emphysema. N Engl J Med 2003;348:2058–73.

Rennard SI. Anticholinergics in combination bronchodilator therapy in COPD. In: Spector SL, ed. Anticholinergic Agents in the Upper and Lower Airways. New York: Marcel Dekker, 1999:119–36.

Russi EW, Imfeld S, Boehler A, et al. Surgical treatment of chronic COPD. *Eur Resp Mon* 2006;38:359–74.

Schenkein JG, Nahm MH, Dransfield MT. Pneumococcal vaccination for patients with COPD: current practice and future directions. *Chest* 2008;133:767–74.

Szafranski W, Cukier A, Ramirez A et al. Efficacy and safety of budesonide/formoterol in the management of chronic obstructive pulmonary disease. *Eur Respir J* 2003;21:74–81.

Tashkin DP, Celli B, Senn S et al. A 4-year trial of tiotropium in chronic obstructive pulmonary disease. *N Engl J Med* 2008;359: 1543–54.

Tashkin DP, Rennard SI, Martin P et al. Efficacy and safety of budesonide and formoterol in one pressurized metered-dose inhaler in patients with moderate to very severe chronic obstructive pulmonary disease: results of a 6-month randomized clinical trial. *Drugs* 2008;68:1975–2000.

Troosters T, Donner CF, Schols AMWJ et al. Rehabilitation in COPD. *Eur Resp Mon* 2006;38:337–58.

The course of COPD, particularly as the disease advances, is associated with episodes of acute increases in symptoms. These flare-ups or exacerbations can last from several days to weeks, and may occur several times a year with varying frequency in different individuals. These debilitating events result in unscheduled visits to healthcare professionals, hospitalizations and, occasionally, a need for ventilatory support and increased mortality.

Acute exacerbations of COPD place a large burden on healthcare resources. It has been estimated that, in an average UK Health Authority with a population of 250 000, there will be 14 200 consultations with a primary care physician and 680 hospital admissions for exacerbations of COPD each year. In the UK, respiratory admissions account for 25% of all acute emergency admissions, and COPD accounts for more than half of these, representing 203 193 hospital admissions in 1994. A UK survey of respiratory units found that 73% of men and 23% of women aged 65–74 years were admitted because of COPD. Recent studies have suggested that up to 50% of patients do not report exacerbations, so the true frequency is much higher than the number of consultations with primary care physicians suggests. Thus, the healthcare burden imposed by exacerbations of COPD is enormous.

Definition

There is no general agreement on the definition of an exacerbation of COPD. Most definitions of exacerbations are based on increasing symptoms and/or increased healthcare utilization. A commonly used definition characterizes exacerbations based on the type and number of symptoms, such as increases in dyspnea, sputum volume or sputum purulence with or without symptoms of upper respiratory infection (Table 8.1). Most studies have defined exacerbations as worsening of symptoms requiring changes in normal treatment, including increased bronchodilator therapy, use of antimicrobial therapy or use of short courses of oral glucocorticosteroids. Recently, an exacerbation of COPD

TABLE 8.1

Definition of COPD exacerbation

Type I

Three of: increased breathlessness, sputum volume or sputum purulence

Type II

Two of: increased breathlessness, sputum volume or sputum purulence

Type III

One of: increased breathlessness, sputum volume or sputum purulence

plus

one of the following symptoms:

- upper respiratory infection (sore throat, nasal discharge) within the past 5 days
- fever without other cause
- increased wheezing
- increased cough
- increase in respiratory or heart rate by 20% compared with baseline

Adapted from Anthonisen et al. 1987.

was defined as 'an event in the natural course of the disease characterized by change in the patient's baseline dyspnea, cough or sputum that is beyond the normal day-to-day variations, is acute at onset, and may warrant a change in regular medication in a patient with underlying COPD'. Fatigue may also be prominent.

The severity of an exacerbation can also be defined in terms of increasing healthcare utilization as: mild (self-managed by the patient at home); moderate (requiring treatment by the primary care physician and/or hospital outpatient attendance); or severe (resulting in admission to hospital). The severity of an exacerbation and the consequent healthcare utilization may depend on the severity of the underlying COPD.

Exacerbations of COPD are characterized by worsening pulmonary gas exchange and increasing hypoxemia (Table 8.2). Respiratory failure may develop in those patients with severe underlying disease or during severe exacerbations. Deterioration in gas exchange is largely due to an increased ventilation–perfusion mismatch. Hypoxemia during an exacerbation of COPD is usually due to increased areas of lung with low ventilation:perfusion ratios. The hypercapnia of respiratory failure, which occurs in some exacerbations, is due to a number of factors including the increased work of breathing resulting from the increase in airways resistance and increase in systemic carbon dioxide production, and respiratory muscle fatigue. Sustained worsening is defined as symptoms worse than normal for at least 24 hours. A staging system for exacerbations of COPD has recently been proposed using clinical descriptors to characterize acute exacerbations (Table 8.3).

Pathophysiology

Pathology studies of exacerbations in COPD have been performed on postmortem material and bronchial biopsies. Recently, inflammation has also been assessed by non-invasive surrogate markers in sputum and breath. Relatively few of these last studies have involved patients with COPD, and patient numbers have been small.

TABLE 8.2

Physiological changes in COPD exacerbations

- Worsening hypoxemia primarily due to an increase in areas of the lungs with a low ventilation:perfusion ratio
- Increased dead space (wasted ventilation) as areas of the lung with a high ventilation:perfusion ratio increase
- Increased resistance to airflow in the upper and lower airways
- Increased work of breathing
- Hypercapnia in patients with underlying severe COPD or during severe exacerbation
- Pulmonary hypertension

TABLE 8.3

Staging of COPD exacerbations based on healthcare utilization

Severity	Level of healthcare utilization
Mild	Patients have an increased need for medication, which they can manage in their own normal environment
Moderate	Patients have an increased need for medication and feel the need to seek additional medical assistance
Severe	Patients/caregivers recognize obvious and/or rapid deterioration in condition, requiring hospitalization

It has been assumed that increased inflammation in the airways is a characteristic feature of exacerbations of COPD. However, the presence of increased inflammation, and particularly the type of inflammation that is present, is controversial and depends on whether the inflammatory response is assessed in sputum, bronchoalveolar lavage fluid or bronchial biopsy, and on the severity of the exacerbation. The few studies of biopsies from patients with exacerbations of COPD have predominantly comprised patients with chronic bronchitis with mild airflow limitation; in some of these studies, increased levels of eosinophils were present in induced sputum and in bronchial biopsies from patients with exacerbations. However, neutrophils are also present in increased numbers in the bronchial walls and in bronchoalveolar lavage fluid in exacerbations of COPD.

Surrogate markers of inflammation, such as sputum levels of tumor necrosis factor α, interleukin (IL)-8 and IL-6, have been shown to be elevated in exacerbations of COPD. Oxidative stress is a major component of the airway inflammation in COPD. Surrogate markers of oxidative stress are known to be elevated, compared with levels in healthy smokers, in the blood, exhaled breath and breath condensate of patients with stable COPD, and are further increased during exacerbations of COPD.

Etiology

The main etiologic factors in exacerbations of COPD are thought to be bacterial and viral infections, and air pollutants. Other factors associated with exacerbations of COPD are social deprivation and changes in temperature. However, in around 30% of exacerbations of COPD, no obvious etiologic factor is found.

Bacteria. Between 30% and 50% of patients with exacerbations of COPD have a positive sputum culture for bacteria. However, around 20–30% of clinically stable patients also have a positive bacterial culture from sputum. Bronchoscopic protected specimen brush biopsies show that bacteria are present in the lower airways in greater numbers during exacerbations than in the stable clinical state, suggesting infection. The main organisms present in sputum in exacerbations of COPD are *Haemophilus influenzae*, *Streptococcus pneumoniae* and *Moraxella catarrhalis*. Gram-negative bacteria, such as *Pseudomonas aeruginosa*, are less common during exacerbations of COPD, but occur with increasing frequency in patients with severe airflow limitation. In some studies, atypical bacterial pathogens such as *Chlamydia pneumoniae* have been found during exacerbations of COPD. Changes in bacterial strain have also been associated with acute exacerbations.

Respiratory viruses. Several studies have shown that viruses are present in around 30% of acute exacerbations of COPD. They are associated with increased inflammation in the airways and a more prolonged time to the resolution of symptoms.

Air pollution is now a well-established cause of exacerbations of COPD. Epidemiological studies show links between the levels of particulate air pollution and emergency admissions for exacerbations of COPD. Other air pollutants, such as ozone, have also been associated with exacerbations of COPD in epidemiological studies.

Natural history
Studies in the 1960s, particularly in the UK, suggested that exacerbations of COPD were associated with small and transient decreases in respiratory function, and therefore did not alter the natural history of the disease. However, this view has recently been challenged, and it is believed there may be a small, but significant, accelerated

decline in lung function as a result of exacerbations of COPD. There are several large population studies showing that the number of exacerbations experienced correlates with the severity of the underlying disease. The median number of exacerbations in patients with severe COPD is around 2.2–2.5 exacerbations per year.

Follow-up of patients with exacerbations of COPD shows a high readmission rate of around 30% over the first 3 months. Patients with recurrent exacerbations (three or more exacerbations per year) have a higher mortality rate and a decreased quality of life.

Symptoms and signs

Patients with acute exacerbations typically present with increased cough, changes in sputum volume and/or purulence, and increased breathlessness, wheezing and chest tightness. The clinical history, examination and arterial blood gases are used to assess the severity of the exacerbation in order to judge whether a patient requires admission to hospital. A number of other non-specific symptoms, such as malaise, sleepiness, fatigue and confusion, may occur in exacerbations. Fever may be present and an increase in sputum purulence suggests a bacterial cause, as does a history of chronic sputum production. The severity of the exacerbation is assessed from the medical history, particularly the severity of the underlying COPD, the presence of pre-existing comorbidities, the physical examination and gas measurements (Table 8.4).

Respiratory failure may or may not be present, as may cyanosis and the flapping tremor of hypercapnia, but these signs are rather insensitive. Pulse oximetry can rapidly provide information about oxygen saturation, but arterial blood gases should be measured in all patients with severe exacerbations. Peak expiratory flow measurements are not as useful for determining the need for hospital admission in COPD as they are in asthma. Chest radiographs may be useful to diagnose conditions that may mimic symptoms of an exacerbation (see pages 120 and 122).

The presence of purulent sputum during an exacerbation is usually a sufficient indication for starting empirical antibiotic treatment. If an exacerbation does not respond to such treatment, sputum should be cultured and bacterial sensitivities identified.

TABLE 8.4

Assessment of severity of COPD exacerbations

History

- Severity of underlying airflow limitation is measured by forced expiratory volume in 1 second
- Duration or severity of new symptoms
- Number of previous episodes (exacerbations/hospitalizations)
- Comorbidities
- Current treatment regimen

Signs of severity

- Use of accessory muscles of respiration
- Worsening or new onset of cyanosis
- Hypercapnia (e.g. flapping tremor)
- Development of peripheral edema
- Reduced alertness

Several conditions may mimic COPD exacerbations including congestive cardiac failure, pneumothorax, pneumonia, pulmonary embolism and cardiac arrhythmia. It is particularly important to consider these differential diagnoses in patients with exacerbations of COPD who do not respond to treatment.

Prevention

Prevention or reduction in the severity or length of exacerbations of COPD is a major goal of management. Influenza vaccination is recommended since it reduces hospitalization for pneumonia in elderly patients with COPD during epidemics. Vaccination against streptococcal pneumonia is available and is effective in preventing the complications of the infection.

There is now evidence that a range of drugs including long-acting β-agonists, inhaled corticosteroids and long-acting anticholinergic agents can reduce the frequency of exacerbations. The combination of a long-acting β-agonist and an inhaled corticosteroid is more effective in reducing exacerbations than either agent individually.

The use of mucolytic agents in COPD has been evaluated in a number of studies. The effects on the frequency of exacerbations have been mixed. There is, however, some evidence that, in COPD patients who have not been treated with an inhaled corticosteroid, mucolytics may reduce exacerbations.

Management

The aims of management in exacerbations of COPD are to relieve airway obstruction, correct hypoxemia, address any comorbid disorder that may contribute to respiratory deterioration and treat any precipitating causes such as infection.

Management at home. Most exacerbations of COPD are treated in primary care; only a minority of patients are admitted to hospital.

Bronchodilators. The dose and the frequency of use of bronchodilators are increased in home management of exacerbations of COPD. If not already used, therapy with multiple bronchodilator classes may be added if symptoms are not improving. In the most severe cases, high-dose nebulized bronchodilators can be given on a regular or as-required basis for several days. However, there is evidence that the use of multiple doses of bronchodilators by metered-dose inhaler with a spacer device has an effect similar to that of nebulized bronchodilators in exacerbations of COPD. When a nebulizer is used, it is probably safer to use air as the driving gas, rather than oxygen, and to continue oxygen therapy via nasal prongs. The long-term use of nebulized therapy after acute exacerbations of COPD is not routinely recommended.

Antibiotics. The use of antibiotics in exacerbations of COPD is still controversial. In mild-to-moderate exacerbations, sputum culture is not usually necessary. Patients with two or more of the following symptoms – increased breathlessness, sputum production and sputum purulence – show greater improvement with antibiotics than with placebo during exacerbations of COPD. Simple antibiotics, modified according to local bacterial resistance patterns, should be used. Amoxicillin can be given in most cases as first-line treatment, or co-amoxiclav in those who fail to respond or who are known or suspected to have β-lactamase-producing organisms in their sputum. Clarithromycin is an alternative in patients who are hypersensitive to penicillins.

Glucocorticosteroids. The use of corticosteroids in exacerbations of COPD is now well established. Several controlled trials have shown that systemic corticosteroids achieve a greater improvement in spirometry, reduced length of stay in hospital and fewer treatment failures than placebo. The exact dose of corticosteroids that should be given has not yet been established, but present evidence suggests that 30–40 mg/day for 7–10 days is appropriate.

Hospital treatment. Provisional guidelines provide indications for hospital admission for acute exacerbations of COPD (Table 8.5).

Blood gases should be measured in all severe exacerbations of COPD. A partial pressure of oxygen in arterial blood (PaO_2) below 6.7 kPa (50 mmHg), a partial pressure of carbon dioxide in arterial blood ($PaCO_2$) above 9.3 kPa (70 mmHg) or a pH below 7.3 suggests a life-threatening episode that needs close monitoring or management in an intensive care unit (ICU).

The presence of a pulmonary embolism, which can mimic an exacerbation of COPD, can be very difficult to diagnose, particularly in patients with COPD. Chest radiographs are useful in diagnosis. A low diastolic blood pressure and an inability to increase the PaO_2 to more than 8 kPa (60 mmHg) despite oxygen therapy also suggest pulmonary embolism. Spiral computed tomography pulmonary angiography is the best tool available for diagnosis of pulmonary embolism. Ventilation/perfusion scanning is of no value in patients with COPD.

The first actions when treating patients hospitalized with an exacerbation of COPD are to provide controlled oxygen therapy and to determine whether the exacerbation is life-threatening, in which case admission to an ICU is indicated. Management of other acute exacerbations of COPD is summarized in Table 8.6.

Oxygen therapy aims to maintain adequate oxygenation (PaO_2 > 8 kPa [60 mmHg] or percentage oxygen saturation of arterial blood [SaO_2] > 90%) without worsening the hypercapnia. Many

TABLE 8.5

Indications for hospital admission for acute exacerbations of COPD

The more referral indicators that are present, the more likely the need for admission to hospital

	Treat at home	Treat in hospital
Ability to cope at home	Yes	No
Breathlessness	Mild	Severe
General condition	Good	Poor and deteriorating
Level of activity	Good	Poor or confined to bed
Cyanosis	No	Yes
Worsening peripheral edema	No	Yes
Level of consciousness	Normal	Impaired
Already receiving long-term oxygen therapy	No	Yes
Social circumstances	Good	Living alone or not coping
Acute confusion	No	Yes
Rapid rate of onset	No	Yes
Changes on the chest radiograph	No	Present
Arterial pH level	≥ 7.35	< 7.35
PaO_2	≥ 7 kPa (52 mmHg)	< 7 kPa (52 mmHg)

PaO_2, partial pressure of oxygen in arterial blood.
Source: British Thoracic Society Guidelines for the management of chronic obstructive pulmonary disease. *Thorax* 1997;52(suppl 5):S1–S28.

patients who have chronic hypoxemia will tolerate a lower PaO_2 (> 6.7 kPa [50 mmHg]) after administration of oxygen. Oxygen is given in inspired concentrations of 24–28% by Venturi mask or 1–2 liters/minute by nasal prongs. Arterial blood gases should be measured to ensure satisfactory oxygenation without additional retention of

TABLE 8.6

Management of severe but not life-threatening exacerbations of COPD

- Assess severity of symptoms, blood gases and chest radiograph
- Administer controlled oxygen therapy – repeat arterial blood gas measurement after 30 minutes
- Bronchodilators
  - increase dose or frequency
  - combine β-agonists and anticholinergic agents
  - use spacers or air-driven nebulizers
  - consider adding intravenous aminophylline, if needed
- Corticosteroids, oral or intravenous
- Antibiotics when signs of bacterial infection are present, given orally or occasionally intravenously
- Consider mechanical ventilation
- At all times:
  - monitor fluid balance and nutrition
  - consider subcutaneous heparin
  - identify and treat associated conditions (e.g. heart failure, arrhythmias)
  - closely monitor condition of the patient

carbon dioxide and consequent acidosis. Oxygen masks provide a more accurate inspired oxygen concentration, but nasal prongs are better tolerated.

Bronchodilator therapy can mitigate the effects of increased airway obstruction, namely increased respiratory work of breathing (hyperinflation, respiratory muscle mechanical disadvantage and impaired ventilation/perfusion matching), causing hypoxemia in patients with exacerbations of COPD. Short-acting β-agonists are preferred as initial bronchodilators in acute exacerbations. Although they are usually given in nebulized form, there is evidence that administration of β-agonists via metered-dose inhaler and spacer device is equally efficacious. Nebulizers should be powered by compressed air rather than oxygen if the $PaCO_2$ is raised, to prevent worsening hypercapnia and acidosis. Oxygen administration via nasal prongs can continue at 1–2 liters/minute during nebulization. If the response to a β-agonist is not prompt, or if the patient has a very severe exacerbation, the anticholinergic drug ipratropium bromide can be added.

The role of intravenous aminophylline in the treatment of COPD exacerbations is controversial. Studies have shown minor improvements in lung volumes following administration of aminophylline, but also worsening gas exchange. Monitoring of serum theophylline levels is recommended to avoid the side effects of these drugs.

Glucocorticosteroids have been shown to reduce symptoms and improve lung function effectively in patients with acute exacerbations of COPD. Currently, systemic corticosteroids, 30–40 mg/day for 7–10 days, are recommended for all patients with an acute exacerbation in the absence of significant contraindications. Oral corticosteroids are preferable. Nebulized budesonide is an alternative to oral corticosteroid treatment in exacerbations without respiratory failure and is associated with a reduction in complications, such as hyperglycemia. Corticosteroids should be discontinued after the acute episode; clinical improvement with corticosteroids during the exacerbation does not indicate the need for long-term treatment with oral or inhaled corticosteroids.

Antibiotic therapy in exacerbations of COPD was the subject of a meta-analysis of nine randomized, placebo-controlled trials. This analysis established a small but significant benefit, which was most evident in patients with the most symptoms. When two of the three cardinal symptoms (increasing breathlessness, increasing sputum volume and increasing sputum purulence) were present, there was a significant improvement following treatment with antibiotics compared with placebo.

In most cases, sputum Gram-stain or culture is unnecessary. Oral rather than intravenous antibiotics should be given. Failure to respond to simple antibiotics (as described above), the known presence of β-lactamase-producing organisms in sputum or severe exacerbations are all indications for a broader spectrum antibiotic, such as co-amoxiclav, a second- or third-generation cephalosporin or fluoroquinolone, or a newer macrolide.

Sputum clearance. Airway inflammation in exacerbations of COPD promotes mucus hypersecretion. There are no convincing data to support the use of pharmacological agents to improve mucokinetics during exacerbations. The use of mechanical techniques such as physiotherapy have no proven value in acute exacerbations, unless a large amount of sputum (> 25 mL) is produced daily or there is mucus plugging with lobar atelectasis. Physiotherapy is not recommended in patients with acute-on-chronic respiratory failure.

Diuretics are indicated in the presence of edema and raised jugular venous pressure.

Anticoagulants, specifically prophylactic subcutaneous heparin, should be administered to patients with severe exacerbations, particularly those who are immobile and those with acute-on-chronic respiratory failure.

Ventilatory support

The objectives of mechanical ventilatory support in patients with exacerbations of COPD are to reduce mortality and morbidity, and relieve symptoms. Ventilatory support includes both non-invasive ventilation using negative or positive pressure devices and invasive mechanical ventilation by endotracheal intubation.

Non-invasive intermittent ventilation has been shown in several randomized control trials in acute respiratory failure in COPD to reduce respiratory acidosis, the severity of breathlessness, the length of stay in hospital, the need for intubation and mortality. Non-invasive ventilation is not appropriate for all patients (Table 8.7).

Invasive mechanical ventilation. The indications for initiating invasive mechanical ventilation during exacerbations of COPD are shown in Table 8.8. Use of invasive ventilation in patients with end-stage COPD is influenced by the patient's wishes and the likelihood of reversing the precipitating events. A clear statement of the patient's own treatment wishes – an advance directive – may make these decisions easier.

TABLE 8.7

Indications and contraindications for non-invasive ventilation

Indications

- Moderate-to-severe breathlessness with use of accessory muscles and paradoxical abdominal motion
- Moderate-to-severe acidosis (pH $\leq$ 7.35) and/or $PaCO_2$ > 6 kPa (45 mmHg)
- Respiratory frequency > 25 breaths/minute

Exclusion criteria

- Respiratory arrest
- Cardiovascular instability (arrhythmias, hypotension, myocardial infarction)
- Change in mental status, uncooperative patient
- High aspiration risk
- Viscous or copious secretions
- Craniofacial trauma
- Nasopharyngeal abnormalities
- Extreme obesity

$PaCO_2$, partial pressure of carbon dioxide in arterial blood.

TABLE 8.8

Indications for invasive mechanical ventilation

- Unable to tolerate or failure of non-invasive ventilation
- Severe breathlessness or respiration rate > 35 breaths/minute
- Life-threatening hypoxemia
- Severe acidosis (pH < 7.25)
- Respiratory arrest
- Impaired mental status
- Vascular complications (hypotension)
- Other complications (metabolic, sepsis, pneumonia, pulmonary embolism)

Hospital discharge and follow-up

There are no data indicating the optimal duration of hospitalization for acute exacerbations of COPD, but suggested discharge criteria are listed in Table 8.9. Follow-up assessment 4–6 weeks after discharge from hospital is recommended (Table 8.10). The presence of hypoxemia during an exacerbation of COPD should prompt rechecking of blood

TABLE 8.9

Discharge criteria for patients with acute exacerbations of COPD

- Inhaled β-agonist therapy is required no more frequently than every 4 hours
- Patient, if previously ambulatory, is able to walk across room
- Patient is able to eat and sleep without frequent disruption by dyspnea
- Patient has been clinically stable for 12–24 hours
- Arterial blood gases have been stable for 12–24 hours
- Patient (or home caregiver) fully understands correct use of medications
- Follow-up and home-care arrangements have been completed (e.g. visiting nurse, oxygen delivery, meal provision)
- Patient, family and physician are confident that patient can manage successfully

TABLE 8.10

Follow-up assessment for acute exacerbations of COPD 4–6 weeks after hospital discharge

- Assess ability to cope in usual environment
- Measure forced expiratory volume in 1 second
- Reassess inhaler technique
- Check patient's understanding of recommended treatment regimen
- Assess need for long-term oxygen therapy and/or home nebulizer (for patients with severe COPD)

gases at discharge. If the patient remains hypoxemic, the need for long-term outpatient oxygen therapy should be assessed when the patient attains a stable state.

Recent randomized controlled trials have shown that 20–30% of patients hospitalized with acute exacerbations of COPD can be safely allowed home with support without adverse consequences.

Key points – acute exacerbations of COPD

- Acute exacerbations of COPD are common and place a huge burden on healthcare resources.
- The main etiologic factors in acute exacerbations are bacterial infection, respiratory viruses and air pollution.
- Treatment includes oxygen, increased use of bronchodilators, antibiotics and short-term oral glucocorticosteroids.
- Exacerbations can be prevented by inhaled corticosteroids and vaccination against influenza.
- Most exacerbations of COPD are managed at home, but those with suspected respiratory failure should be admitted to hospital.
- Non-invasive ventilation has been shown to reduce mortality in patients with acute-on-chronic respiratory failure.

Key references

Anthonisen NR, Manfreda J, Warren CPW et al. Antibiotic therapy in exacerbations of chronic obstructive pulmonary disease. *Ann Intern Med* 1987;106:196–204.

Davies L, Angus RM, Calverley PMA. Oral corticosteroid in patients admitted to hospital with exacerbations of COPD: a prospective randomized trial. *Lancet* 1999;354:456–60.

MacNee W. Acute exacerbations of COPD. Consensus conference on management of chronic obstructive pulmonary disease. *J R Coll Phys Edinb* 2002;32:1–46.

Niewoehner DE, Erbland ML, Deupree RH et al. Effect of systemic glucocorticoids on exacerbations of COPD. *N Engl J Med* 1999;340:1941–7.

Rodriguez-Roisin R. Towards a consensus definition for COPD exacerbations. *Chest* 2000;117: 398S–401S.

Saint S, Bent S, Vittinghoff E, Grady D. Antibiotics in chronic obstructive pulmonary disease exacerbations. A meta-analysis. *JAMA* 1995;273:957–60.

Seemungal TAR, Donaldson GC, Bhowmik A et al. Time course and recovery of exacerbations in patients with COPD. *Am J Respir Crit Care Med* 2000;161:1608–13.

Seemungal TAR, Donaldson GC, Paul EA et al. Effect of exacerbation on quality of life in patients with COPD. *Am J Respir Crit Care Med* 1998;157:1418–22.

Siafakas NM, Vedzicha JA. Management of acute exacerbation of COPD. *Eur Respir Mon* 2006;38:387–400.

New therapies in development

Research in the area of COPD is vigorous, and current investigations are shedding new light on its pathogenesis. Advances in our understanding of the mechanisms responsible for the lung damage and the systemic aspects of COPD will enable new therapeutic targets to be identified (Table 9.1). Because of the high prevalence and burden of COPD, there is a correspondingly large potential market. The pharmaceutical industry has responded with major investments in exploring novel therapeutic targets, and a number of new agents are under investigation.

TABLE 9.1

Targets for novel therapies for COPD

Pro-inflammatory signaling
- Cytokines
- Cytokine receptors
- Cytokine receptor signaling pathway components

Inflammatory mediators
- Proteinases
  - serine
  - metalloproteinases
  - cysteine
- Oxidants
- Defensins
- Complement
- Injury pathways
  - apoptosis
  - cell adhesion factors

Neural pathways
- Modulator pathways
- Transmitters
- Receptor agonists/antagonists

Repair
- Growth factors
- Differentiation factors
- Stem cells

The first such agents to reach clinical practice may be phosphodiesterase-4 inhibitors, which have both bronchodilator and anti-inflammatory actions.

Improved understanding of disease

Recent improvements in our understanding of COPD are likely to lead to more sophisticated diagnostic and therapeutic approaches. Recognition that dyspnea is an inspiratory event and that dynamic changes related to respiratory rate are major contributors is likely to lead to improved physiological assessment of the COPD patient. Improvements in imaging technology, including high-resolution computed tomography (CT) scanning and magnetic resonance imaging, hold great promise for better defining the anatomy of the lung of the COPD patient; CT scanning is now mandatory before lung-volume reduction surgery. Multiple dimensional assessments that incorporate physiology together with performance measures, symptom scores and other domains have proved highly useful in clinical trials. Investigation of similar measures in clinical practice is now under way. Improved methods to evaluate exacerbation frequency, severity and duration will improve both clinical trials and clinical management.

Improved methods of diagnosis

Fundamental changes in the way COPD is approached are also likely to change clinical practice. To date, COPD has been defined simply, and a diverse group of patients with a heterogeneous collection of conditions has been grouped together. Treatments at present are symptom-based and attack common mechanisms shared by most patients. It is probable that, in the near future, more sophisticated diagnostic methods will be applied to identify subsets of patients who respond to more mechanistically based treatments. Such treatments may be much more effective than current therapies, albeit for a smaller proportion of patients. It may be that COPD will become fragmented into many conditions, each of which may include only a small group of patients. This approach holds particular promise for modifying the progressive nature of the disease.

Potential for lung repair

Strikingly, recent studies have demonstrated that the lung has considerable capacity to repair itself following injury. In animal models, emphysema can be reversed by the administration of all-*trans*-retinoic acid (Figure 9.1). Similar studies are currently under way in humans to evaluate the use of agents selective for the retinoic acid receptor. Clinical trials with mesenchymal stem cells, which may have both anti-inflammatory effects as well as the potential to mediate repair, are under way. The possibility that lung function can be restored in COPD patients is particularly exciting.

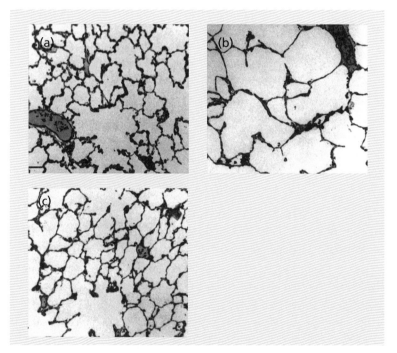

Figure 9.1 Rat lung alveolar regrowth after treatment of elastase-induced emphysema with all-*trans*-retinoic acid (ATRA). (a) Control. (b) Tissue after instillation of elastase. (c) Tissue from a rat with elastase-induced emphysema after treatment with ATRA. Reproduced with permission from Macmillan Publishers Ltd © 1997, from Massaro GD, Massaro D. Retinoic acid treatment abrogates elastase-induced pulmonary emphysema in rats. *Nature Med* 1997;3:675–7.

Prevention of COPD

The most important future direction, however, is prevention of COPD. Recognizing the risk factors for COPD, particularly cigarette smoking, makes this eminently feasible. Advances in preventing people from starting to smoke and in promoting cessation among established smokers could not only slow the progression of existing COPD, but also prevent new cases developing. Recent data from the USA demonstrated a decrease in mild airflow limitation among younger Americans in conjunction with a reduction in smoking initiation and prevalence (Figure 9.2), which may herald a downward slope of the COPD epidemic.

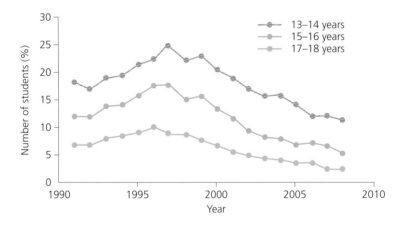

Figure 9.2 Smoking behavior of young people in the USA. Data from Johnston LD, O'Malley PM, Bachman JG, Schulenberg JE (December 11, 2008). *More good news on teen smoking: rates at or near record lows.* Ann Arbor: University of Michigan News and Information Service, 2008. www.monitoringthefuture.org

Useful addresses

UK

British Lung Foundation
73–75 Goswell Road
London EC1V 7ER
Helpline: 08458 50 50 20
www.lunguk.org

British Thoracic Society
17 Doughty Street
London WC1N 2PL
Tel: +44 (0)20 7831 8778
bts@brit-thoracic.org.uk
www.brit-thoracic.org.uk

QUIT
*UK site for smokers who want to
stop*
63 St Marys Axe
London EC3A 8AA
Tel: +44 (0)20 7469 0400
Quitline: 0800 00 22 00
info@quit.org.uk
www.quit.org.uk

Quitnet
*US site for smokers who want to
stop*
www.quitnet.com

USA

American Association for
Respiratory Care
9425 N MacArthur Blvd, Suite 100
Irving, TX 75063-4706
Tel: +1 972 243 2272
info@aarc.org
www.aarc.org

American College of Chest
Physicians
3300 Dundee Road
Northbrook, IL 60062-2348
Tel: +1 847 498 1400
Toll-free: 1 800 343 2227
www.chestnet.org

American Lung Association
1301 Pennsylvania Ave, NW
Suite 800, Washington, DC 20004
Tel: +1 212 315 8700
Helpline: 1 800 548 8252
www.lungusa.org

American Thoracic Society
61 Broadway
New York, NY 10006-2755
Tel: +1 212 315 8600
www.thoracic.org

Professional Assisted Cessation Therapy (PACT)
Materials for clinicians, including research updates
c/o RSi Communications Group
118 Main Street
Tappan, NY 10983
pact@endsmoking.org
www.endsmoking.org

Respiratory Nursing Society
c/o Donna Bond, Treasurer
309 E Lee Avenue
Vinton, VA 24179
MaFnds@aol.com
www.respiratorynursingsociety.org

International
Action on Smoking and Health (ASH)
www.ash.org.uk (UK)
www.ash.org (USA)
www.ashaust.org.au (Australia)

European Respiratory Care Association
www.eurorespicare.com

European Respiratory Society
4, Ave Sainte-Luce
CH-1003 Lausanne, Switzerland
Tel: +41 (0)21 213 0101
info@ersnet.org
www.ersnet.org

Global Initiative for Chronic Obstructive Lung Disease
(includes GOLD guidelines)
www.goldcopd.com

International Primary Care Respiratory Group
Samantha Louw
Centre of Academic Primary Care,
Foresterhill Health Centre
Westburn Road, Aberdeen
Scotland AB25 2AY, UK
Tel: +44 (0)1224 552427
http://theipcrg.org

The Lung Association (Canada)
1750 Courtwood Crescent, Suite 300
Ottawa, ON K2C 2B5, Canada
Tel: +1 613 569 6411
Toll-free: 1 888 566 5864
info@lung.ca
www.lung.ca

The Thoracic Society of Australia and New Zealand
145 Macquarie Street
Sydney, NSW 2000
Australia
Tel: +61 (0)2 9256 5457
admin@thoracic.org.au
www.thoracic.org.au

Index

What the reviewers say:

"This concise, up-to-date, well-illustrated text represents excellent value for money . . . it's unique in being able to pack so much relevant information into such a small volume, which makes it highly readable"

British Medical Association,
on *Fast Facts – Minor Surgery*, 2nd edn,
(First Prize, Primary Health Care, BMA Book Awards 2008)

"This short textbook provides a quickstop guide to STIs . . . it's handy for both medical students and allied healthcare professionals"

British Medical Association,
on *Fast Facts – Sexually Transmitted Infections*, 2nd edn
(Commended, Public Health Care, BMA Book Awards 2008)

"An outstanding up-to-date compilation of facts on psoriasis, a must-read for any healthcare provider with an interest in psoriasis, whether casual or in-depth"

Dr Gerald Krueger, Professor of Dermatology, University of Utah School of Medicine,
on *Fast Facts – Psoriasis*, 2nd edn, Jan 2009

"A very accessible summary of the key facts about lymphoma, presented in clear language with straightforward explanations"

Leukemia Research Fund,
on *Fast Facts – Lymphoma*, Oct 2008

"A useful addition to this well-known series . . . very affordable and excellent value for money"

ICS News, Feb 2008
on *Fast Facts – Bladder Disorders*

"Buy it for yourself . . . but be careful your colleagues don't borrow it indefinitely"

on *Fast Facts – Asthma*, 2nd edn
Primary Health Care, July 2007

www.fastfacts.com